P9-BYR-605

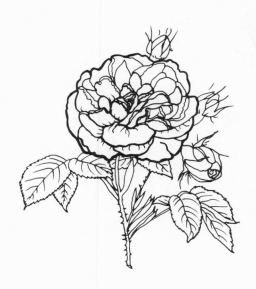

With Love to

From

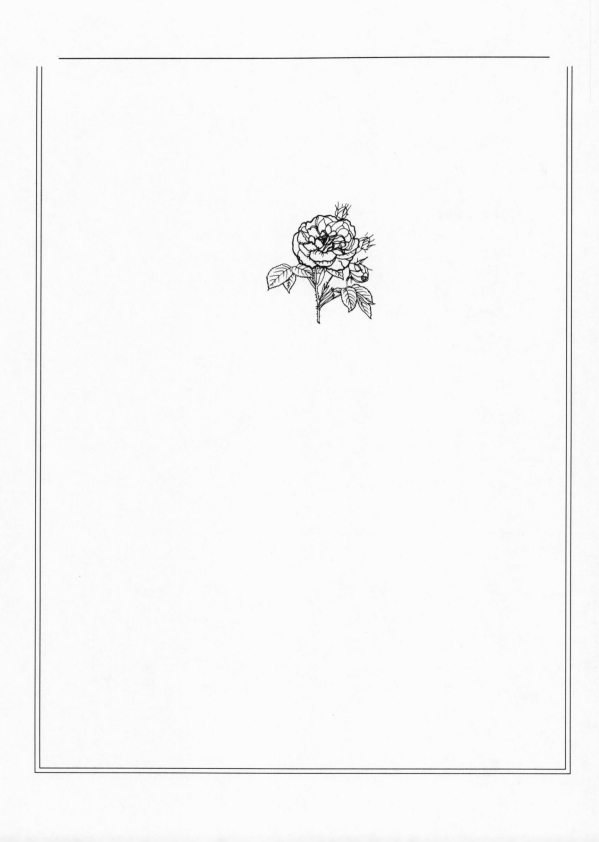

ROMANTIC MASSAGE

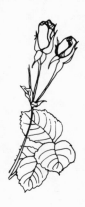

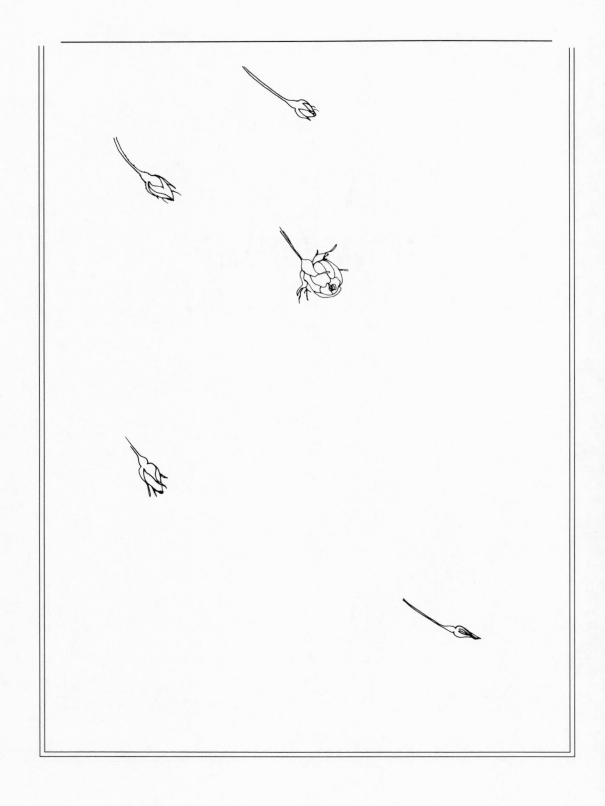

ROMANTIC MASSAGE

Ten Unforgettable Massages for Special Occasions

ANNE KENT RUSH

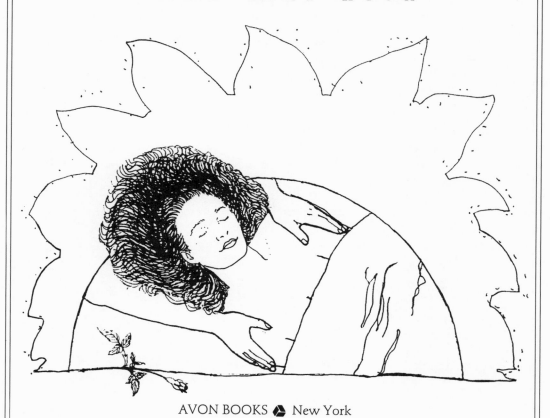

AVON BOOKS ◆ New York

Romantic Massage is an original publication of Avon Books. Published by arrangement with the author. This work has never before appeared in book form.

AVON BOOKS
A division of
The Hearst Corporation
105 Madison Avenue
New York, New York 10016

Special thanks to my editor, Judith Riven; agents, Katinka Matson and John Brockman; cameraman, Laurence Singer; typesetter, Maura Balliett; and models who asked to remain mysterious.

Text and illustrations copyright © 1991 by Anne Kent Rush
Library of Congress Catalog Card Number: 90-22277
ISBN: 0-380-75985-3
Typeface: Schneidler

All rights reserved, which includes the right to reproduce this book or portions thereof in any form whatsoever except as provided by the U.S. Copyright Law. For information address John Brockman Associates, Inc., 2307 Broadway, New York, New York 10024.

Library of Congress Cataloging in Publication Data:

Rush, Anne Kent, 1945–
    Romantic massage : ten unforgettable massages for special
occasions / Anne Kent Rush.
    p. cm.
    1. Massage.   2. Intimacy (Psychology)   3. Interpersonal relations.
I. Title.
RA780.5.R874   1991   90-22277
613.9′6—dc20   CIP

First Avon Books Trade Printing: February 1991

AVON TRADEMARK REG. U.S. PAT. OFF. AND IN OTHER COUNTRIES, MARCA REGISTRADA, HECHO EN U.S.A.

Printed in the U.S.A.

ARC   10   9   8   7   6   5   4   3   2   1

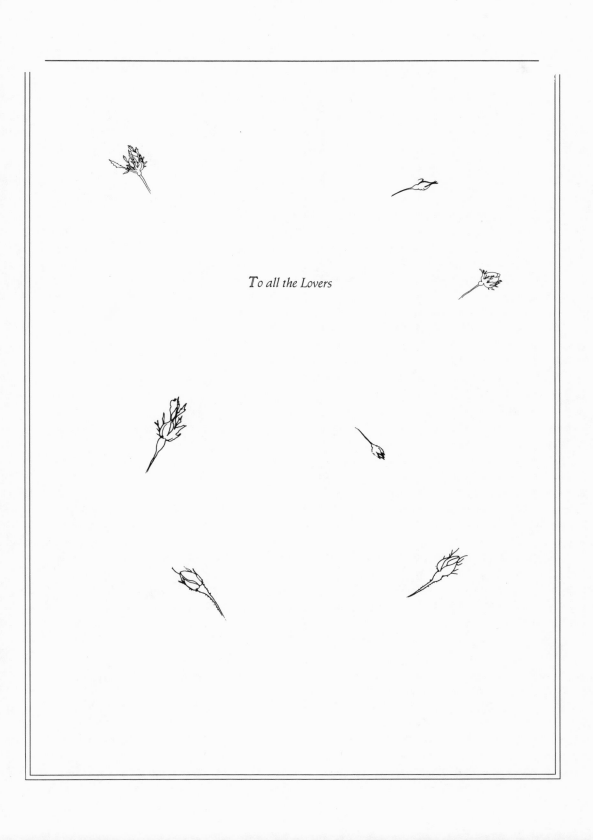

To all the Lovers

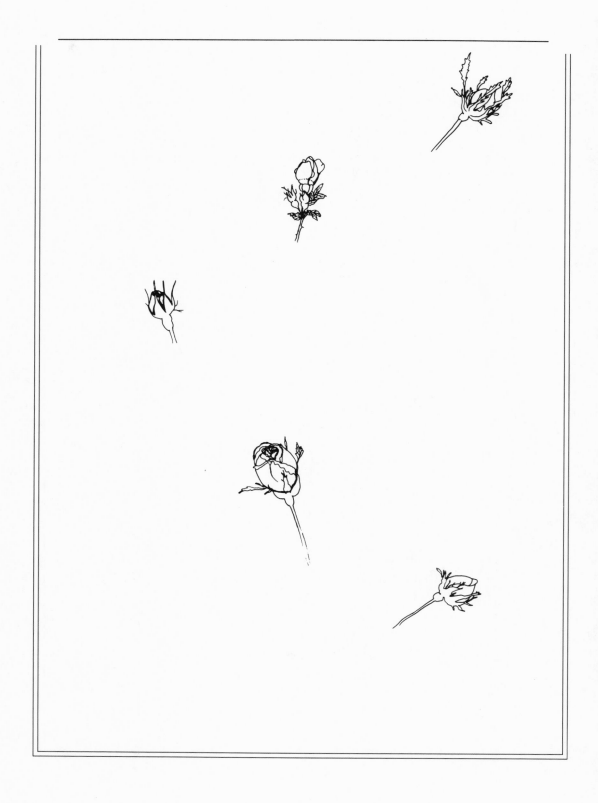

Contents

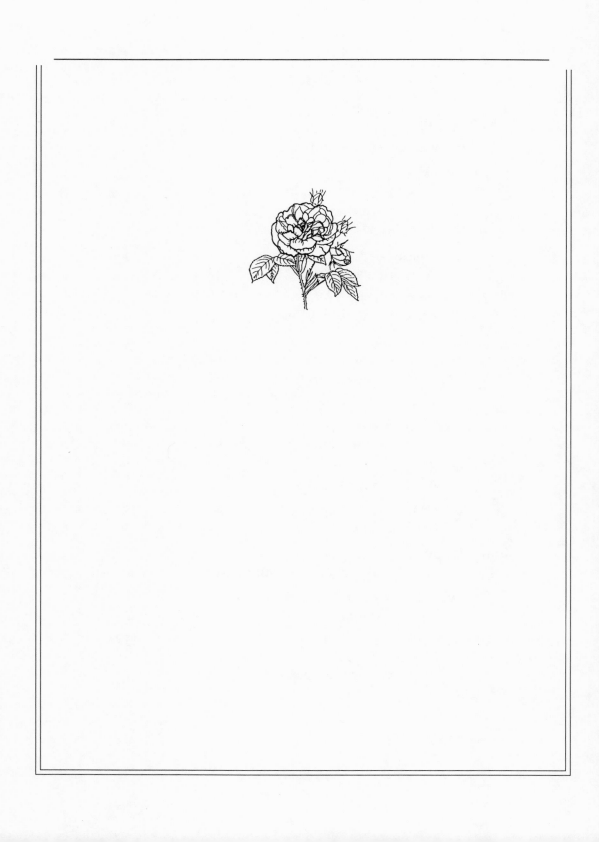

ROMANTIC MASSAGE

What is this thing called love?
Cole Porter

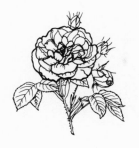

I

Love in Mind

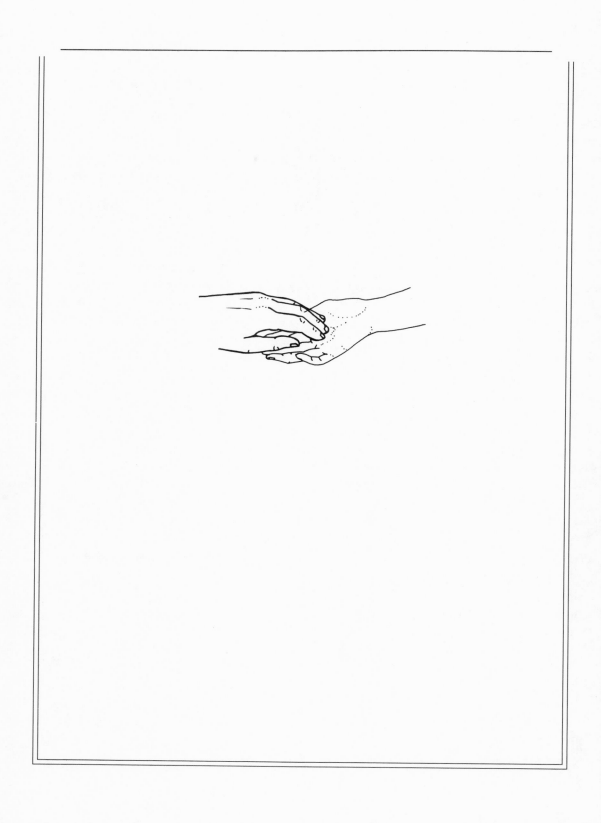

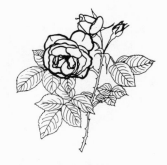

The Touch of Your Hand

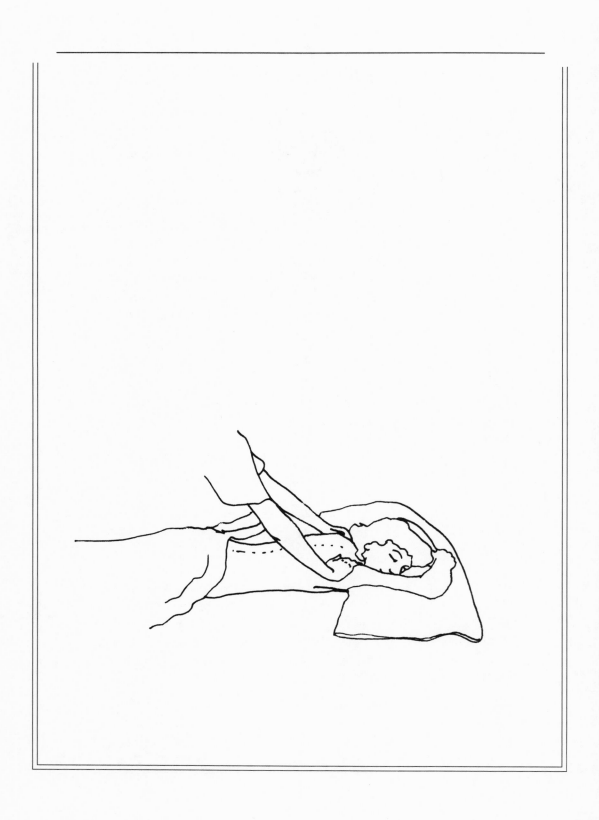

The Touch of Your Hand

We all love to be touched with tenderness. Infants love touch. We hug our friends. We caress our lovers with special warmth. A loving touch is like no other; it exhilarates and renews the giver and the receiver.

You can say some things non-verbally that you can't say verbally. If you want to say I love you with intensity. If you want to affirm that you care for someone's comfort and wellbeing. Even when you want to say I'm sorry. You can express these feelings beyond words with a touch. Central to romance is the desire for the touch of your loved one's hand. More thrilling than anyone's touch, the touch of your lover can change a moment into paradise now, becoming an unforgettable memory.

Simple acts of caring are often the most exciting part of romance. The phone call when it wasn't expected. The touch of your loved one's hand in a crowd of strangers to remind you of a shared private world. The flowers that arrive on your unbirthday. The love letter that comes in the mail from someone you live with. The back rub after a hard day at the office. The foot rub after a long hike. The full massage just to make you feel good.

Romance is these happy surprises that make us forget our everyday worries. Romance is feeling appreciated and pampered. Romance is sharing moments of pleasure with someone you love.

Communication in the world of romance is largely non-verbal, and it is here that massage is most delightful. Massage heightens your body sensitivity and expands the scope of communication with loved ones. This book presents a bouquet of complete massages that are events in themselves to show how massage can lead the way to romance. And who can resist a little romance?

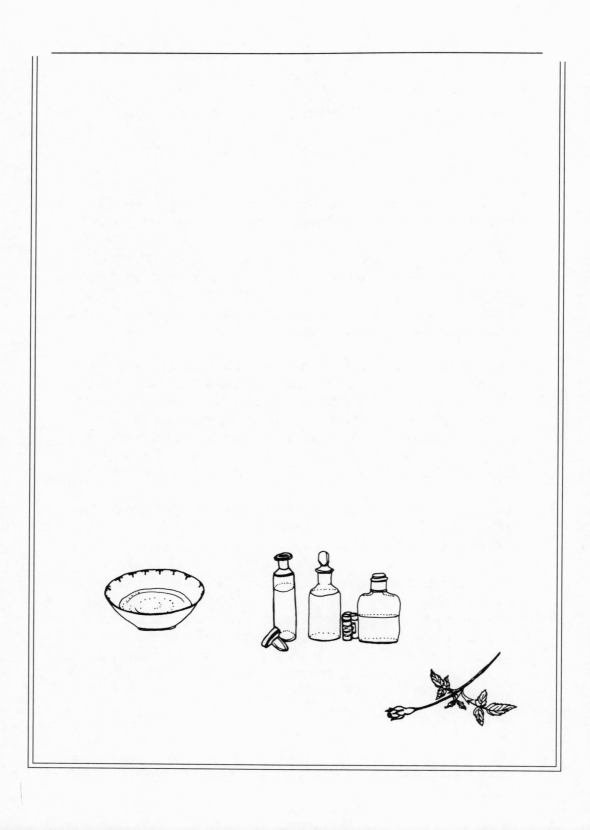

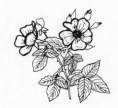

Fundamental Things to Apply

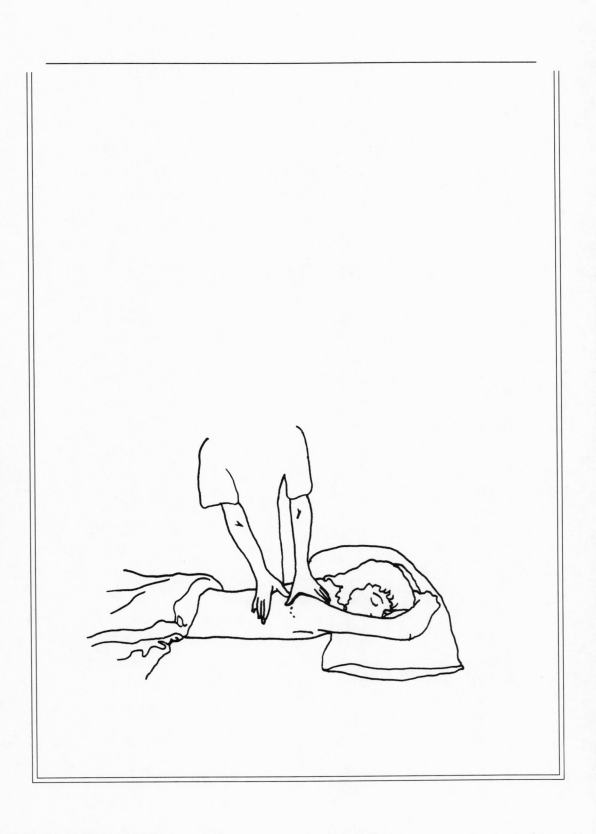

Fundamental Things to Apply

You can give a great romantic massage. All you need are love, good instincts and some oil. However, variety is a spice of romance, and as time goes by you'll probably want to expand your repertoire. The massages in this book offer suggestions on some different kinds of body treats you can share with your lover.

Each romantic massage is focused on a different mood. Most are short. This means you can learn a massage quickly and incorporate it easily into your schedules. When you and your lover have a luxurious stretch of unhurried time, you can also combine two or more of the short massages to create a long one. Or simply repeat each stroke in a short massage ten or more times. A good stroke feels better the more you do it and as you both relax. But even a little massage goes a long way. So don't worry if you don't have a lot of time. Ideally massage would be part of each day. Wouldn't it be lovely?

Simple Things Mean A Lot

Most of the techniques in these massages are purposely simple. Your focus for a romantic massage should not have to be on mastering complicated strokes, but on expanding your own sensual expression and communication. The basic strokes described in these chapters are to be tailored to you and your lover's tastes. The pressure the two of you like, the rhythms and speeds you prefer, the favored ways your fingers cup your lover's curves—these qualities can not be dictated by a text, but their discovery can be made inevitable by massage.

It Takes Two

Though there is no formula guaranteed to produce a fine romance, you can create conditions that give romance the best chance to bloom. The massages described here do not depend on certain settings, fixed agendas or sexual involvement for success. Romance builds on a mysterious combination of spontaneous

5

combustion and mutual attraction. You know long before you touch that you want to be close. Massage can be part of your tentative contact before you are lovers and part of your romance in different ways during different phases of your friendship and affair.

If You Believe in Me

When asked, "What is romantic?" most people agree on some basic ingredients. Like excitement, romance is a feeling; you know when it's there and when it's missing. Like magic, romance imbues an ordinary event with special meaning that gives it power. Drinking a glass of orange juice can be as romantic as splitting a bottle of champagne if you're sharing it at a particularly happy moment.

I've interviewed a varied cast of lovers and incorporated their suggested pleasures into these massages. These are the sets and props. You and your lover provide the central magic—the openness to explore something new together, the excitement of discovering mutual desires.

The Way You Do the Things You Do

The basics of a good therapeutic massage are easily available: some fragrant vegetable oil; a comfortable quiet setting; a relaxed giver;and a willing receiver. What takes this pleasant experience beyond relaxation into romance?

Add elements to your massage that will show that you've paid attention to your lover's tastes and that you enjoy indulging them. If he or she is a nature lover, try the picnic or beach massage. If you're making overtures to a musician, choose one of their favorite pieces to accompany your massage. Bring some of your lover's favorite flowers for the room, and some of their favorite foods. Name a massage after them. Such touches show you cherish their individuality, and this is the essence of romance.

For most of us, the experience of having our needs and tastes catered to for an extended time is a luxurious treat. The intensity of attention heightens the romantic feeling.

While giving a massage, if you let your mind wander and are just going through the motions, the receiver can feel the lack of focus. This emotional distance can be fine in a therapeutic massage but it's not particularly romantic. During the massage, focus on your non-verbal, sensual communication. Give yourself over to the responses of your partner's body and to your own pleasure in touching. The receiver feels this attention, and it enhances the romantic mood between you.

Bridge Over Work Day Waters

In romance, massage can become a bridge to help you cross from a hectic day into the special realm of romance. At the close of a stressful work day or week, a great back rub can do a lot to wipe away tension and leave you and your lover revived. Most of us need a transition to help our minds stop spinning on the day's problems and turning to relaxation and sensuality. Massage can provide this for both of you. Massaging someone you love before you make love will probably heighten their sensitivity and inspire them to be a more sensual lover.

Timing Tells

Love and romance take time to cultivate. Carving out intimate moments with your lover is essential to continuing the process. The length of time you take is not necessarily the key to how romantic it is. A long massage is divine. A short massage, a brief respite in your hurried schedule, can also be extremely romantic.

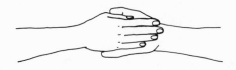

Receiving and Giving

Initiating a romantic massage is sometimes emotionally risky for both the receiver and giver. The receiver has more responsibility for the success of a romantic massage than for a therapeutic one. If you are receiving the massage, you'll want to communicate your likes and dislikes but be sure to express them in a friendly, encouraging way. Sensitivity to criticism runs higher during a romantic massage than during other kinds. Happily, praise carries more weight also. The most reliable rule of etiquette is to phrase your dislikes in terms of specific preferences. Rather than, "Don't press so hard," saying, "I like lighter pressure. Could you try that?" gets the message across without criticism and with a clear alternative.

Hopefully the receiver will be interested in discovering fresh sensations and will enjoy the massage in a light, open mood. Romance and making love are creative processes. Part of the fun is learning things about yourself and your lover. Massage is almost always a window to new non-verbal communication.

Giving a romantic massage offers you the opportunity to be more playful than a regular massage. Dream up treats and surprises for the event. Giver as well as receiver should have a good time.

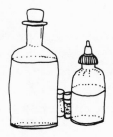

Oils and Aromas

An effective massage can be given even when the receiver is clothed. The material provides a substitute for the oil so the masseur's hands can slide without scraping the skin.

Receiving a romantic massage, you are most likely to be nude and using oil. Massage oil makes all sorts of strokes possible that otherwise would be uncomfortable because of friction. Any vegetable oil such as sunflower, safflower or almond, makes a wonderful massage oil. Avoid peanut unless you want to smell like one.

Oil also opens the door to the exploration of scent. Aroma therapy is a system that correlates certain scents with specific emotional states. You and your lover can have fun with this by selecting the scent for the massage oil together, according to which mood it evokes in you. Some vials of essential scent oils are sold at many drug stores and cosmetic shops. Just a few drops of oil of mint, almond, cinnamon or musk will scent a whole jar of massage oil.

Using oil and firm pressure usually eliminates any tickling your partner might feel. If the tickles persist, just move to another area to massage.

Aphrodisiacs, Potions and Food

Food and drink often function as strong aphrodisiacs. Feeding your partner is an integral part of every animal's courtship ritual. Massage (and romance) can be physically tiring, so it's always delightful to have some refreshing treats nearby. Light fare is important. Massage on a full stomach is not comfortable. A glass of lemonade and a sandwich after a beach massage or a hot toddy before your goodnight massage can be the perfect additions.

If your partner has special food cravings, cater to them. Additionally there is much lore about aphrodisiac foods. Oysters and seafood have long been eaten as sexual stimulants. Ginseng root bolsters the body's nervous system and was prized by Chinese emperors as the key to ongoing sexual vitality. Chocolate contains substances which trigger the body's natural opiates. Foods not generally thought of as aphrodisiacs become so because of your shared associations with them.

A very useful guide for lovers' meals is *The Yachting Cookbook* by Wheeler and Trainer (Crown, 1990) because the scrumptious gourmet fare is designed to be made quickly and usually served as picnics.

You're Getting to Be a Habit With Me

Equally as exciting as initiating a romance is the skill of continuing the seduction and exploration throughout the developing relationship. To keep romance alive you'll need to start with fireworks and proceed to revive the spark over time. For a true romantic, courtship is continuous. Because much of lovers' communications take place on a non-verbal level, massage provides pleasurable access to this realm. As you and your lover accumulate a private history together, you can enjoy reminiscing about especially exciting or loving events. These tales become a delightful part of your language of romance. Lovers have their own histories and calendars. You can make any day Valentine's Day with a romantic massage.

10

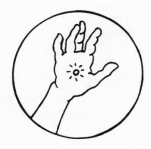

Palm Centering

Visualization can be used to affect your body and your basic
massage technique. Try visualizing pleasurable sensations being
focused during a massage, and you may find your mind is one of
your most erotic organs. This exercise is for channeling energy
through your hands.

Sit either on the floor, or on a chair with your feet on the ground
(legs uncrossed), spine comfortably erect. Relax your hands palms
up in your lap. Allow your breathing to settle low in your abdomen until you can feel your belly move in and out as you exhale
and inhale. Try to clear your thoughts and relax any tense
muscles.

Imagine that as you inhale, your breath moves down your torso
into your belly; as you exhale it moves up through your torso into
your arms. Imagine how it would feel if your exhalation could
move down through the center of your arms as your circulation
does.

Imagine that each time that you exhale your breath moves
farther down the inside of your arms until it reaches your hands.
Send your breath out through a spot in the center of your palms
about the size of a coin. Can you feel the breath moving out
through this spot? (A variation is to feel the energy moving out
through the fingers.)

Now keeping your arms relaxed, raise your hands off your lap. Hold them close but not touching, palms facing. Continue exhaling out your palms. Focus on the space between your two palms. Do you feel anything happening between them?

Move your hands slowly apart, paying attention to the space between your hands as you do. Does the sensation change with distance? Now move them toward each other. How does the closeness feel?

Now let your hands move as they want to. Try not to think of things to do but allow the motion to come from your hands. How would they like to move now? At what distance apart and in what position are they most comfortable? Play. Experiment with different movements and positions, tuning in to any sensations you might feel between them as they move.

Now let your hands rest in your lap again. Tune in to anything you may be feeling in your arms, torso or other parts of your body as a result of this exercise.

Slowly open your eyes. Can you stay with the new feelings in your hands and arms even when your eyes are open?

This exercise gives you a chance to feel some of the sensations of channeling your energy in your body. You could probably feel something (heat, vibration, magnetism, streaming, relaxation) in your arms and hands from this exercise. Someone else could receive this energy into their body by making contact with you when you are relaxed and focused. In a simple way this is the mobilization and exchange of healing energy. Physical and emotional tension block it. Relaxation, vitality and centering increase it. Exchange of it is one of the excitements of touching and being touched with love.

You can learn to increase your ability to channel energy through your hands so that your romantic massages feel especially warm and healing. You can channel this energy throughout your entire body so that all your physical contact becomes more charged.

What are your charms for¿
What are my arms for¿
Use your imagination.

Sung by Ray Charles and Betty Carter

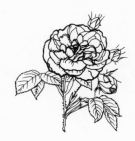

II
The Massages

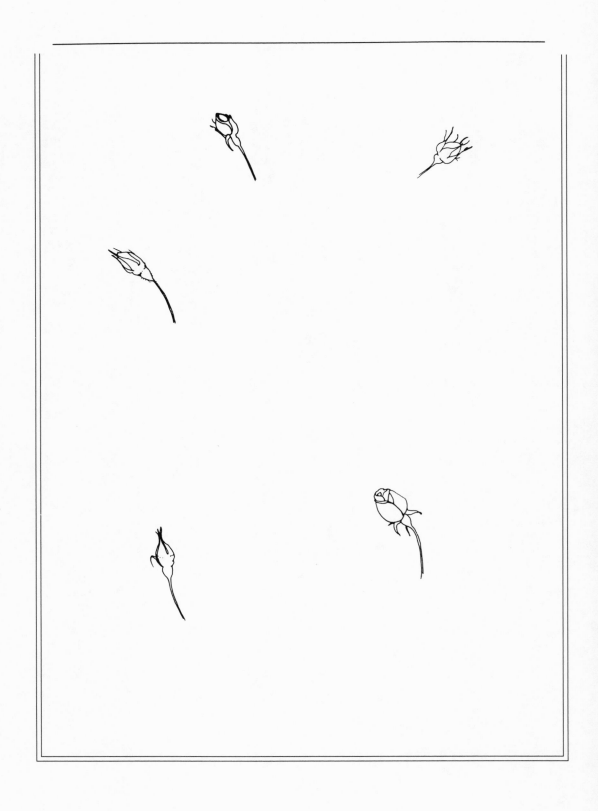

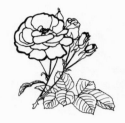

Breakfast in Bed Massage

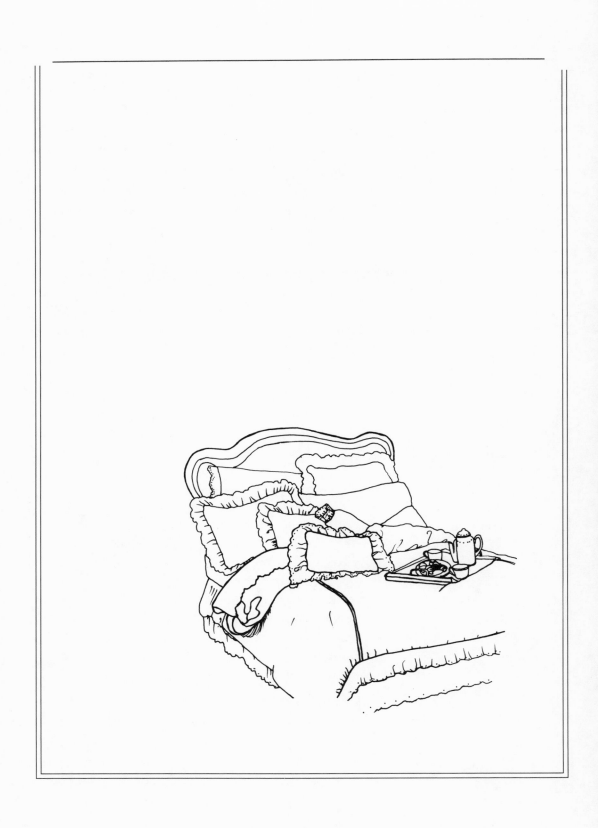

Breakfast in Bed Massage

Greet the Day Refreshed

If you want to be your lover's sunshine, start the day with a good morning massage. If your lover is like Irving Berlin and hates to get up in the morning, he will appreciate being gently soothed into awakening. And a morning massage will make a sensual impression on your love that can keep him or her thinking of the nearness of you all day.

An especially pleasant morning massage is a facial massage. Makes you glad to open your eyes. And the excess oil can be conveniently washed out of your hair and off your face in a morning shower.

Include some neck and shoulder massage as well as scalp massage in your morning facial. Many people experience some neck stiffness in the morning, and the strokes can smooth it away. Scalp massage is helpful in the morning as it is invigorating and improves circulation to the brain to stimulate your mental faculties for the day ahead.

Talking little or not at all is recommended during a morning massage. I'm a firm believer that if someone really loves you, they won't ask you to communicate before breakfast.

Oil is good for the hair and scalp but not necessary for a pleasant head massage because the hair makes sliding over the scalp possible without uncomfortable friction. Almond oil makes a light, lovely face massage oil. My favorite lubricant for face massage is night cream. Very little oil is necessary for face massage. Face cream has plenty and won't clog the pores as some oils can. Morning massages will make you and your love wake up smiling.

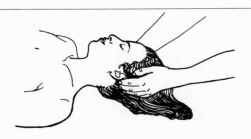

A Loving Facial

15 Minutes

Scalp Rub

Forehead Waves

Third Eye Waves

Eye Glide

Cheekbone Slide

Lip Slides

Ear Sculpting

Chin Sweeps

Full Face Sweep

Neck Slide

Eye Rest

A Loving Facial

Only the perfect Jeeves or a perfect angel is divine enough to appear in the morning with breakfast on a bed tray. Try rising early some morning to prepare your lover's favorite breakfast. Preface this delightful good morning with a sensual scalp and face massage and they'll be convinced you're heaven sent.

Scalp Rub

Relax your hands and try "breathing into your palms" to warm them. Begin by placing your palms lightly on your lover's head and stroking the scalp from the forehead to the back of the head, then down the sides of the head. This is a gentle way to begin massage on a sleepy love and will allow them time to grow accustomed to your touch.

Now lift the head slightly and roll it to the left onto your left palm. Cup your right hand in a claw shape and rub the scalp with your fingertips moving in tiny circles. Press firmly enough that the skin moves a bit over the bone rather than only sliding your fingertips across the surface. Cover the right side of the scalp. Roll the head into your right palm and repeat the stroke with your left hand on the other side of the head.

Forehead Waves

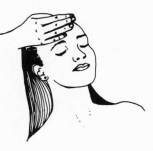

Cup your fingers and palm across the forehead. Press and draw your whole hand up toward the hairline. Lift the hand and begin stroking with the other palm, returning the first hand to continue the stroke. This mimics the motion we often make to wipe away our own forehead tension and is soothing to have done by someone else.

Third Eye Waves

With alternating, overlapping strokes, draw first one thumb and then the other up the bridge of the nose between the eyes and onto the center of the forehead. You can press quite firmly on this bony area. This is a frown area and it relieves tension to massage it. Continue the overlapping strokes ten or more times. This can release sinus pressure. The center of the forehead is the meditation third eye thought to house spiritual sight.

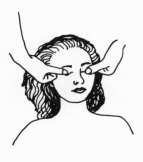

Eye Glide

This stroke is for the eyes themselves and assumes you know your lover is not wearing contact lenses. Gently run the balls of your thumbs straight across your friend's closed eyelids. Start on either side of the nose and move outward. Go slowly. Use a very light pressure. Glide your thumbs out toward the temples. Then lift and return them to the starting point.

Cheekbone Slide

Place the tips of the forefinger and middle finger on each hand to either side of the base of the nose. Press firmly. Draw the fingertips around the lower edges of the cheekbones toward the ears. Then glide up to the temples for circles with your forefingers there. For a variation, glide your fingers to the hinge of the jaw on either side of the face and make firm, deep circles there with your fingertips.

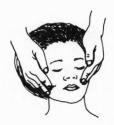

Lip Slides

Place the tips of your forefingers and middle fingers just under the nose and above the mouth. Stroke outward across the cheeks, ending with circles on the jaw hinges. Next do a series of similar strokes across the lips with very light pressure. Start each time at the center and end on the cheeks.

Ear Sculpting

With the tip of your forefinger lightly trace the crevices of the inside of the ear, moving from the outside toward the center, stopping short of closing off the ear channel. Next press your forefinger behind the ear where it meets the head. Then draw your finger up the "V" formed by the topmost part of the ear and the skull.

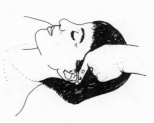

Chin Sweeps

Place the fingertips of both hands facing each other under the chin. Lift gently upward under the chin and press your full fingers against the chin and neck. Slide your hands away from each other in semicircular sweeps out toward the ears. Lift your hands and return to the center under the chin to begin the sweep again.

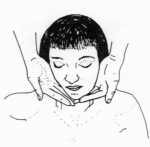

Full Face Sweep

Cup your palms over the face, heels of the hands on the forehead and fingertips resting over the cheekbones. Lean and press down slightly as you slide your hands apart over the sides of the face and down the bed on either side. Lift your hands and return to center to begin the stroke again. Downward pressure

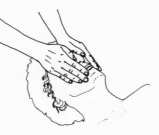

toward the chin is not pleasant or good for the face muscles. Be sure to angle your stroke out and slightly up.

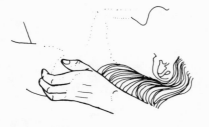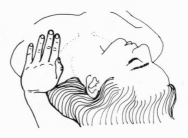

Neck Slide

Slide your hands under the back of your lover's head to raise it slightly. Turn the head gently to the left until it rests in your left palm. Press the fingers from the base of the ear down the muscles along the side of the neck. When you reach the shoulder, press the heel of your right hand onto the top of the shoulder. Circle and press your fingertips around the shoulder and onto the back. Move your fingers across the back muscles toward the spine. Just before reaching the spine, pull your fingers up onto the back of the neck. Continue up the neck muscles until your fingertips reach the base of the skull. Then turn your hand so that your fingers point up and you can glide the hand back down the side of the neck. Continue and repeat the stroke several times.

Eye Rest

Slightly cup both palms and place them over your lover's closed eyes. Rest them in this position a few minutes, allowing both of you to relax. This gesture creates a gentle closing to your massage. Gradually raise your hands off the face. You can lightly seal it with a kiss.

Let your lover rest a bit longer
while you arrange the breakfast tray.

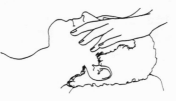

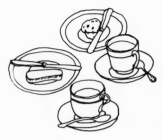

Breakfast in Bed

Coffee or tea, in a thermos to keep very hot

Cream and sugar

*Bowls of fresh cut sections of oranges, figs and raspberries
mixed with johnny jump-up blossoms*

Croissants, muffins or bagels, in a covered dish to keep hot

Strawberry cream cheese

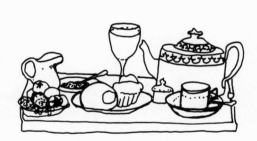

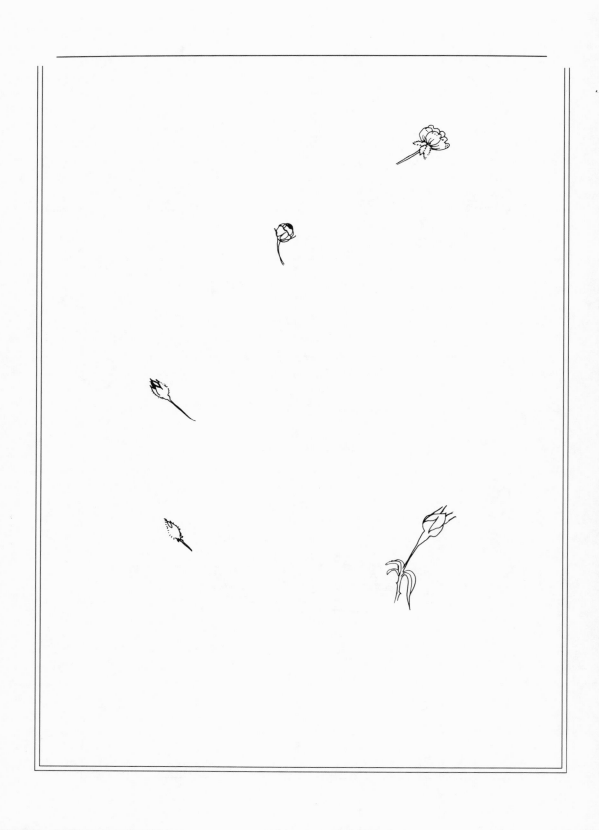

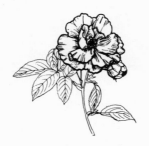

Fireside Massage

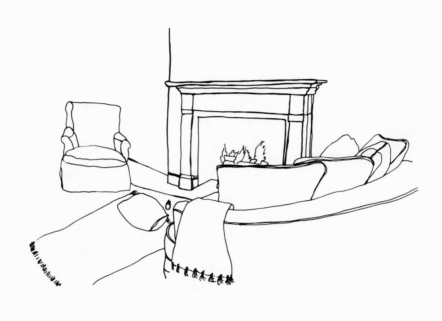

Fireside Massage

Warm a Frosty Winter's Afternoon

Do you want to warm your lover's heart? A fireside massage should make their temperature rise.

Gathering around a fire or hearth creates an emotional as well as a physical warmth. Throughout history people have built fires when they wanted to feel safe. A fireside is a place to dream, to see visions in the flames, to reflect on moments from the past, and to imagine pleasures to come. You can roast chestnuts on the fire. Or you can burn love letters meant for your eyes alone. Sitting by the fire invites storytelling, personal revelations, and perhaps proposals.

Baby, It's Cold Outside

Melt the ice with a fireside massage.

Fireside Massage

20 minutes

Upper Back Circles

Trapezius Squeeze

Palm Slides

Thumbs Along the Spine

Main Stroke

Braided Sweeps

Spine Sweeps

Neck and Sacrum Circles

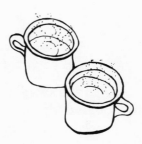

Fireside Massage

If the room is chilly, make sure the fire is roaring and perform the massage with your partner clothed. Even through winter woolens, this back rub can feel fabulous.

Ideally you have preheated the room to a toasty temperature so your partner can be nude and you can massage with oil, a sensual experience in front of a blazing hearth. Before applying the oil, pour in your palm and rub your hands together to warm it. Position yourself so you can both watch the fire.

Prepare a comfortable massage area. If the rug is thick simply use a beach towel covered by a sheet. An exercise or beach pad will cushion a hard floor. You'll need pillows under your partner's head and ankles and one on which you can kneel or sit. Make sure the fire is well stacked so it will last through the massage. You can replenish it before your fireside picnic.

Upper Back Circles

Place your palms on your friend's back and make large, slow circles on their upper back and shoulders.

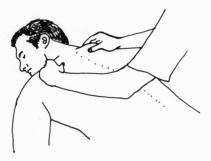

Trapezius Squeeze

Knead the shoulder muscles curving from the neck onto the shoulders. Working the muscles between the thumb and fingers of each hand, do both sides at once. Start with light, slow

squeezes and gradually speed up and squeeze harder; then slow
down again.

Palm Slides

Leaning onto the back from beside him or
her, begin slow, alternating slides with your
palms across the back. Fingertips pointing
away from you, drag one hand toward you
as the other moves away, then reverse.
Make the slides all the way across the back
and sides so the fingertips of one hand
touch the floor opposite you as the heel of
the other hand touches the floor near you.

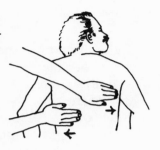

Thumbs Along the Spine

Starting between the shoulder blades, massage the long muscles
on either side of the spine with small circular motions of your
thumbs. Work down to the lower back, up, and down again.
Use deep or light pressure, as your friend prefers. Angle the balls
of your thumbs in between the vertebrae, pressing from the
muscle columns in toward the spine, as though separating the
vertebrae as you massage.

Main Stroke

This stroke covers the whole back thoroughly. Sit beside or on your partner's hips
and work from the waist to the shoulders
and back again. Place your palms on either
side of the waist, heels of the hands on the

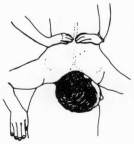

sides, fingers pointing toward the spine but not on it. Slide your hands up the whole back. Maintain firm pressure, leaning forward onto your arms, pressing extra hard with your fingertips so they press into the furrow to either side of the spine as they move.

When you near the top of the spine, separate your hands. Pivot them so your heels are now on either side of the spine and move them across the shoulders and the sides of the torso toward the hips almost hard enough to move your partner toward you. Before reaching the hips again pivot your fingers toward the spine again to repeat the stroke.

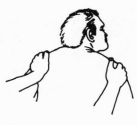

Braided Sweeps

This stroke is usually done with deep pressure. Try it with light pressure as a tantalizing closing to your massage. Place your right hand on your partner's right side of the waist and your left hand on the left side. Slowly pull and press both hands, heels first, toward the spine. When the hands are about to meet, pivot them so that the fingers point toward each other. Moving at the same pace, glide your left hand to your friend's right side and your right hand to the left side. Your forearms will form an X as your hands pass over the spine. Your fingertips will reach the floor pad.

Drawing your hands a little farther up the back, begin the crossing sequence again. Make your way up and down the back in a smooth, continuous motion. Start with a very slow rhythm; gradually speed up; then slow down again.

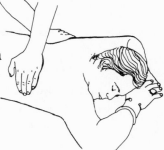

Spine Sweeps

Place your palms on your partner's shoulders. Draw your hands along the muscles on either side of the spine, down the back and over the hips. As you cross the waist, speed up, angle your hands away from each other and finally lift them off the body. Return your palms to the shoulders and begin the sweep again with light, swift strokes.

Neck and Sacrum Circles

Sit to your partner's left. Place your left palm on the base of your partner's neck and your right palm on the sacrum (the triangular bone at the base of the spine). Make slow circles with both palms.

Next simply keep your hands in place a few moments as you imagine you are sending your breath energy down your arms, through your palms and into your partner's back. Very gradually raise your hands off the body while continuing your palm breathing. This is a warm finale to your fireside massage.

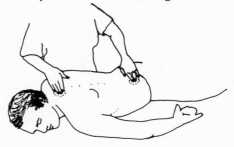

Allow your partner to relax while you arrange the fireside picnic.

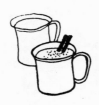

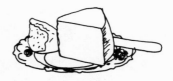

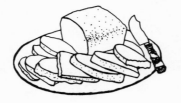

A Fireside Supper

Mulled Wine or Hot Spiced Cider

Smoked Salmon

Leeks Vinaigrette

Canadian White Cheddar and Homemade Brown Bread

Ginger Pound Cake

Fresh Pears

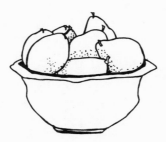

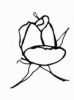

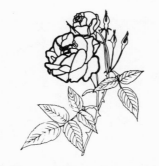

Slow Dancing

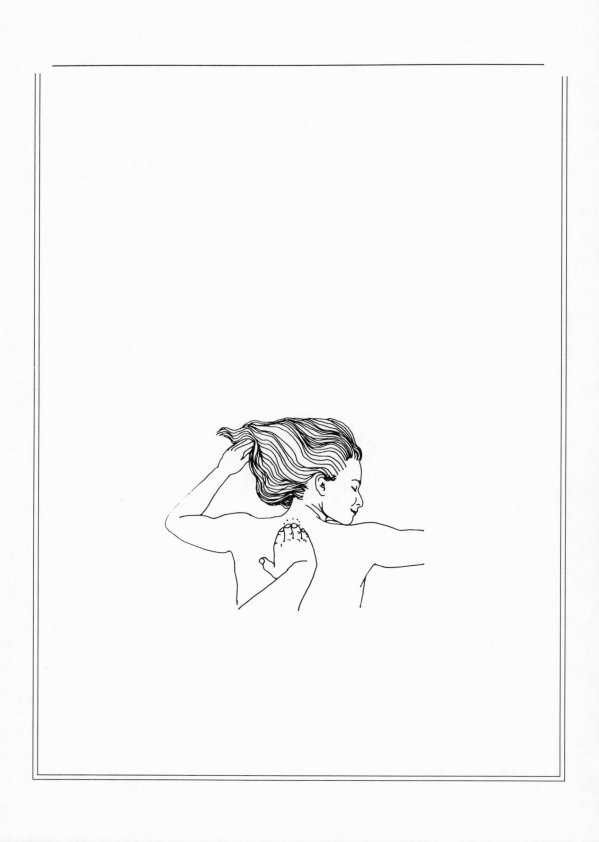

Slow Dancing

Let Music Lead the Way to Romance

Are you in love with a music lover? Improvise a great massage to one of their favorite pieces, and they'll be singing your praises over and over again.

I rarely massage to music because the music imposes its mood and tempo onto the massage. But because it gets you under its spell, massaging to music is highly conducive to invention.

Music can inspire a masseur to invent new strokes and lead you in a surprisingly romantic massage. Each of us has our own habitual pace and pattern of physical movement. If you relax your hands and move to the music's rhythm, you're likely to be led into fresh patterns.

You and the Night and the Music

It's preferable to massage to instrumental rather than vocal music to maintain the non-verbal focus of massage. Music can soothe a sophisticate as well as a savage. And there are times when you may want your mood to be overpowered by outside stimulus.

Move your hands to the music. Let your whole body respond so that the pressure, pace and direction of your strokes vary with your responses to the music. Be sure the music you choose is agreeable to your partner. For a special treat try your dancing massage in the dark.

You're Easy to Dance With

Massaging to music will teach you about planning a massage
well. Many musical pieces are structured the way a good
massage is. A slow beginning to orient the listener. Some
detailed patterns on specific themes. A gradual build-up of
pace to an interesting climax. Then a slowing down of pace
to the closing which repeats original themes to tie it all together. Many good massages start slowly, pick up pace,
include detailed work in the middle and close with whole
body strokes that give the receiver a sense of physical connectedness.

Poetry in Motion

The structure and function of a body part will suggest new
massage strokes. Look at some anatomy charts to familiarize
yourself with the human muscle and bone patterns. As you
massage, angle your stroke in the direction that the muscle
moves and outline the bones. Having one's shape defined by
touch is a reassuring and pleasant part of massage. A good
massage gives the receiver a positive sense of his or her body
shape and of his or her connectedness with the rest of the
environment. After receiving a good massage you'll probably
notice your movements are easier and more fluid from this
physical awareness.

Change Partners and Dance with Me

Feedback is an important part of invention. Your partner
should let you know what feels best and worst.

Receiving good massages also helps you learn how to give
them. Remind your partner that the more massages they give
you, the better yours will be to them.

Though It's Called Dancing, To Me It's Romancing

Here are some suggested improvisation exercises for inventing massages and for simply enjoying the night and the music and the company:

○ Choose a title and then invent the massage to go with it. The Gardener's Special; The Computer Programmer's Delight; The Birthday Surprise.

○ Try giving a massage in a hot bath. Bath oil or soap makes good massage oil. Water invites your hands to move smoothly. Being immersed in hot water while receiving a massage is deeply relaxing.

○ Experiment with massaging to music you'd normally consider little suited to a massage. (*Bolero? Blue Suede Shoes? Hard Day's Night?*) Trying to work with it will force you to do something new. You may not ever want to massage to that accompaniment again but you'll learn something about turning stress into relaxation and take some new strokes away to apply to calmer soundtracks.

○ Give a massage with another masseur or masseuse. It is a terrific and fun way to broaden your repertoire. See the *Two on One* chapter for details.

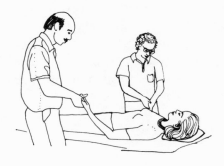

- Do a long half or one hour massage dedicated only to the most neglected areas of the body: arms, knees, back of the neck, ankles, calves. Though they are trickier areas to massage than large areas such as the back or the legs, attention there is wonderful to receive.

- Spend an hour or more on one place only—the back or chest and stomach. With so much time to devote to one area you'll develop details and fine points.

- Use a part of your body you haven't enlisted before to do a massage. This will require new movements and techniques. Elbows are handy for pressure point massage. Forearms feel good for long strokes on the legs or back. Some lovers love having their back stroked with your hair or with your tongue.

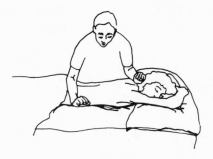

- Decide you're going to only massage in one geometric design, such as circles or straight lines or triangles, and see what movements you discover.

- Let your partner give the orders. Do a whole massage completely directed by your partner's instruction on pressure, timing and strokes.

- Try giving pick-me-up massages while your partner is sitting up or lying on their side or in other new positions.

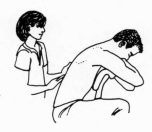

- Choose two of your favorite strokes and limit yourself to these to cover the whole body. This will require you to adapt the strokes to new contours and to combine aspects of each in new ways. Variations will naturally occur.

- Don't fret over precise form or possible mistakes as you improvise. Faux pas can turn into delicious inventions.

To err is human, but it feels divine.

        Mae West

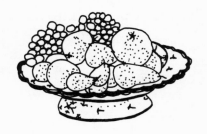

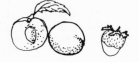

Improvised Meals

Spontaneity is one of the delights of romance. To be elegantly ready for surprise events, your cupboard should stock staples including:

Mineral water, wine, coffee, tea,

Eggs, cheese, spices, crackers, jams,

Frozen bread and muffins,

Fresh fruit

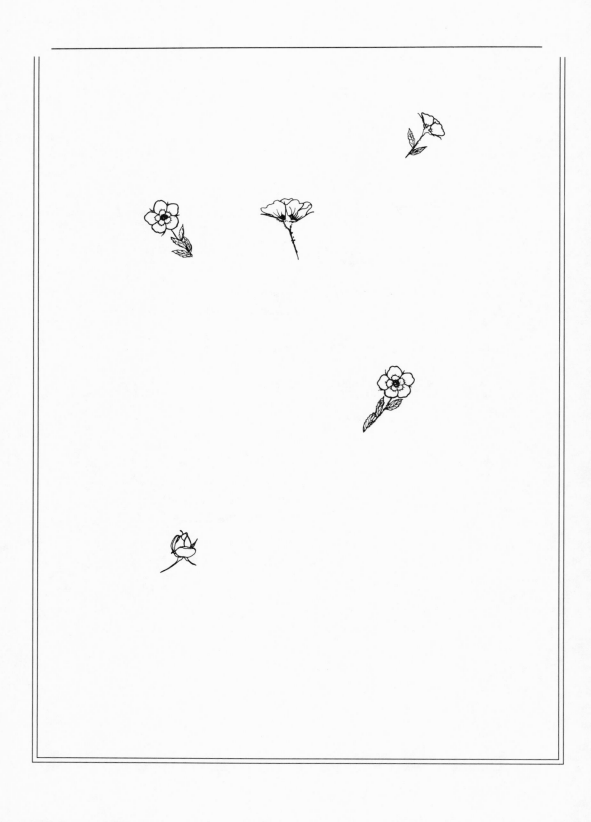

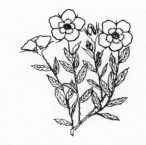

On the Beach

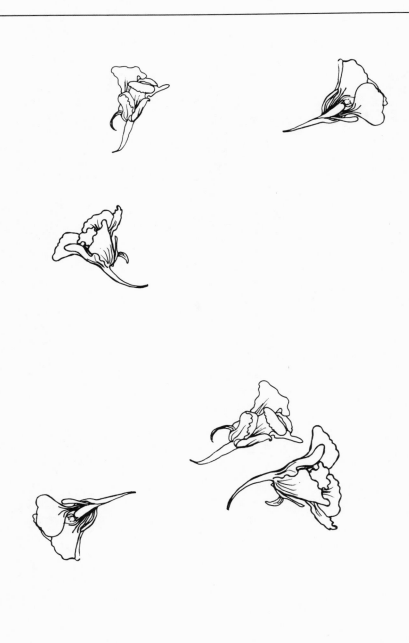

On the Beach

The Best Back Rub Under the Sun

You're on a beautiful beach. The object of your affection asks you to put sun lotion on his or her back. Don't pass up the delightful opportunity to transform a routine act into a romantic interlude. The basic massage ingredients come with the territory: soft place to rest, beach towel, bare back and body lotion. Here's a sun oil application to remember.

On The Beach

10 minutes

Main Stroke

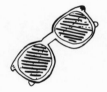

Overlapping Thumbs

Fans and Circles

Spine Snake

Tracing the Spine

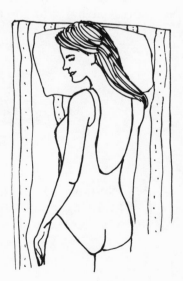

Main Stroke

Sit above your friend's head. Position your palms to either side of the top of the back, with fingers pointing toward the spine and fingertips right beside, but not on, the vertebrae.

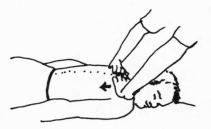

Slide your hands down the whole back. For firm pressure lean forward to make use of your weight.

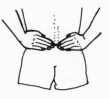

When you near the waist, spread the hands apart and down the sides until they touch the ground. Then slowly pull your hands along the sides of the torso up toward the shoulders.

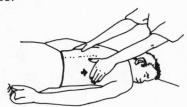

Just before the armpits, bring your hands to the top of the back. Pivot the fingers toward the spine so that they are in place to begin the stroke again.

Overlapping Thumbs

Slide your thumbs away from you in short, fast, alternating strokes. Concentrate on the muscles above the shoulder blades on the shoulders and on the muscles between the blades and the spine.

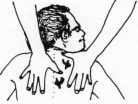

Fans and Circles

Place your palms on the shoulders with your fingers pointing in toward the spine. Leaning onto your hands for pressure, briskly pivot your fingers away from each other in a fanning motion. Then pivot the heels of your hands so the fingers face the spine again. Each fan stroke should slide you a bit down the back. Alternate the fans with full circle strokes in which your whole palm keeps body contact when the fingers pivot back toward the spine. Work all the way down the back several times.

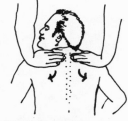

Spine Snake

At the top of the back squeeze and lift the skin over the spine with your thumbs and forefingers. Begin a rolling motion, by sliding your thumbs toward your knuckles, that you will continue all the way to the tailbone. By this point in the massage, some of the oil on the back has been absorbed. That's good because the Spine Snake is easier to do when the back is not very slippery. When you gently grasp a fold of skin, roll it along all the way down to the end of the spine. On the receiving end, this is very releasing because it feels as though nerves are lifted thus relieving pressure from the spine. Try to make the stroke continuous by lifting the next area of skin before completely letting go of the first. This will feel as though you are making one long roll along the whole spine.

Tracing the Spine

With your two forefingers or thumbs, trace the spine from neck to tailbone. Start at the base of the skull. Press moderately with the tips of the fingers letting your fingers curve around vertebrae as you go.

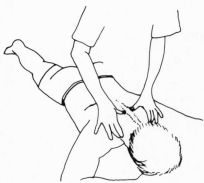

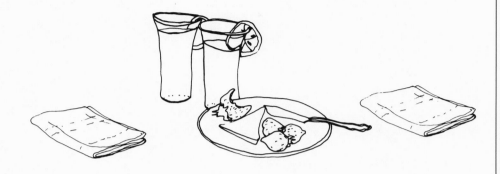

A Beach Picnic

Cold Lemonade in a thermos

Sandwiches of ham, watercress, sundried tomatoes,

nasturtium flowers and mustard

Grapes

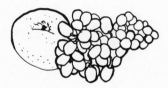

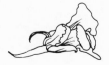

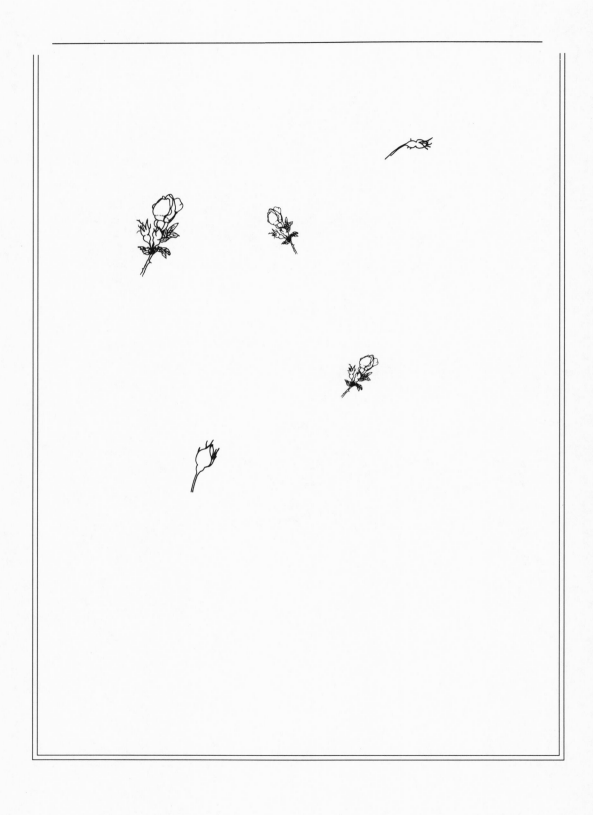

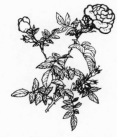

Stress Relief Massage

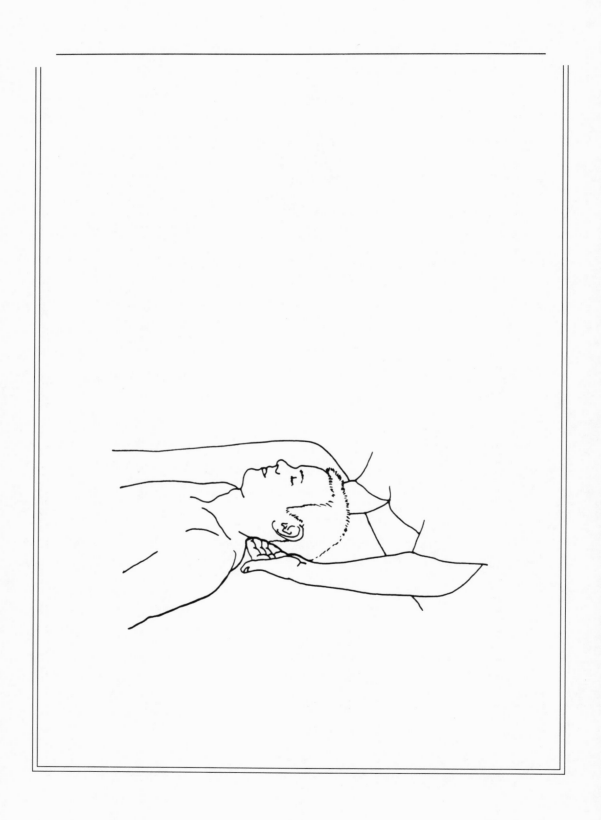

Stress Relief Massage

Rub Away Tension

Romance can be the cause of a great deal of stress. When you say potayto and he says potahto. When you've had quarrels and parted. When you love so much it hurts you. When your lover just can't behave. When you're loco de amor. When you think it was just one of those things. When you're ordering orange juice for one. When you're sure it was just one of those nights. When it keeps raining all the time. When it's your turn to cry over him. When you're just friends.

Whether you're recovering from a Satan in pants or the double crossing of a pair of heels. Or you're fighting vainly the old ennui, a massage may be just what the doctor ordered.

This section offers stress relief exercises to be done with a partner. There are also massage techniques you can do on your lover to revive body, heart and soul.

If you're ready to change your plan and call the whole thing off, make a truce and try a massage. Often after a good massage, every care is gone and you'll call the calling off off.

Stress Relief Massage

20 minutes

Eye Points

Neck Points

Shoulder Points

Foot Points

Lower Back Points

Spine Stretch

Spine Feathers

Stress Relief Massage

Stress from many sources can interfere with romance. You might want to surprise your love with the present of a shiatsu (or pressure point) masseur appearing at his or her office to administer a tension relieving treatment on the job. For reliable references, ask a friend who knows massage professionals. Or call the American Massage Therapy Association at (312) 764-AMTA or contact On Site Massage Association at (800) 678-OSMA.

You can exchange effective stress relief treatments with your lover at home using the following pressure point techniques.

Eye Points

With the tips of both forefingers press up against the bony rims of the eye sockets where they meet the nose. Gradually increase your pressure. Press quite hard for about one full second. Slowly release the pressure and then move about a quarter of an inch along the upper half of each rim to press again. This is good for sinus and headache relief. Continue in this pressure pattern until you have reached the point of each eye socket farthest from the nose. Then return to the point nearest the nose. Begin working the length of the lower half of the rim with this same pressure sequence.

Neck Points

The occipital ridge is the bony shelf at the base of the skull. It houses nerves and tendons from the head, neck, eyes and face. Releasing tension here can relax all those areas.

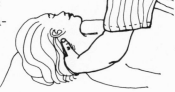

Move to the right side of your partner's head. Lift the head gently with your left hand. Place your right hand under the neck. Your wrist should be at right angles to your arm and should be positioned against the base of your partner's neck. Your fingers will naturally be pointing up your friend's neck toward the occiput.

You want to eventually lower the head onto your thumb and forefinger so that your fingers are pressing into the occiput and the head is resting on them as on a fulcrum. Place your thumb under the occipital ridge on the right side of your partner's spine and your index finger in the matching place to the left of the spine. Very slowly roll and lower the head onto your fingers. When the head is in position, move your left hand from under the skull, and rest it lightly on the forehead. When the weight of the head presses onto your fingers, the area may feel sore at first. Stay with the position. When your friend gets accustomed to the pressure and relaxes the neck some more, the soreness will gradually disappear, and your partner's head will relax back over your fingers onto the table.

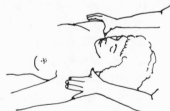

Shoulder Points

Stand above your friend's head. Resting your palms lightly on either shoulder, use both thumbs to apply gradual pressure along the trapezius muscle running from the neck to the outer edges of the shoulders. When you find a spot on the muscle that feels tight and hard, spend more time there to relieve the tension. Pressure should be applied very gradually until you reach a level where you want to be still and hold for a while. When you release the pressure, do it as gradually as you applied it. Don't hurt your friend; this causes tension in the muscle. Apply pressure up to the point of soreness. Then wait for your friend's muscles to relax and soften and move on to the next spot.

Foot Points

Nerves connected to points all over the body make their ways to the feet. Reflexology is a treatment of foot massage based on the theory that you can ease tension or illness in a body part by massaging its corresponding spot in the foot. Refer to the reflexology charts for these correspondences. Whether or not you are treating a specific pain, deep massage all over the foot is greatly relaxing. Use your thumbs to apply pressure all over the soles and sides of the feet.

Lower Back Points

Your partner rolls onto the stomach for this treat. The sacrum is the triangular bone at the base of the spine. Stand beside your partner's hips. Lean your weight into your arms as you press your thumbs on either side of the highest sacral vertebra at the waist. Gradually angle more of your weight into your hands. Release the pressure as gradually as you applied it. Then move your thumbs down beside the next sacral vertebra. Apply the pressure of your body weight and then release. Work your way from the top of the sacrum to the tip. The pressure should be deep but not too painful to your partner. If it is painful, you are pressing either too quickly or too hard for her or him to relax with the pressure. You might not be in quite the right spot, so shift your position and try another spot until the pressure is comfortable.

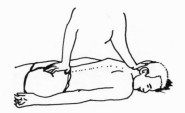

Spine Stretch

While lying facedown your partner's head should be facing away from you to the left. Standing to your partner's right side, take the heel of your right hand and lodge it under the occipital ridge (the base of the skull). Take the heel of your left hand and place it on the sacrum (the triangular bone at the base of the spine), with your fingertips pointing toward the left hip. Gently and gradually apply pressure to the heels of both hands, angling them outward so that you are stretching your partner's spine from top to bottom by pressing the head and sacrum in opposite directions. Release the pressure gradually.

Spine Feathers

This stroke will connect the separate strokes you've done. Place your palms on your partner's shoulders as he or she is lying on the stomach. Draw your fingertips along the muscles on either side of the spine down the back and over the hips. As you cross the hips, angle your hands away and lift them off the body. Return the palms to the shoulders and begin the sweep again with light, swift strokes. Repeat several times.

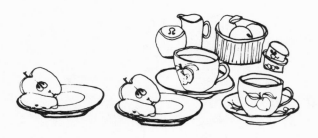

Anti-Stress Snack

Hot chamomile or rose hips teas in winter

Iced mint or lemongrass teas in summer

Honey and lemon

Currant biscuits with Brie cheese

Sliced apples

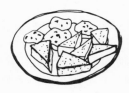

Meditation

Many people think of meditation as a mental exercise. Ideally it is not; it is a way to open yourself to the deepest happenings in your body, and to allow these events to become part of your everyday consciousness. When I keep a routine, just a few minutes each morning and a few minutes each evening changes the quality of my day.

Meditation is an experience which brings to light parts of ourselves on which we do not normally focus. While visualization requires concentration on specific images, meditation asks you to eliminate any visual pictures or thoughts which cross your mind. The easiest way to facilitate this is to concentrate on breathing.

Sit down comfortably erect. Stay focused on your breath rhythm and count to ten, counting each inhalation and exhalation as one unit. Then start counting to ten again. As thoughts come in, let them pass through instead of focusing on them. Let your attention be with your breathing. After awhile the mental static which usually jumbles the mind during the day will clear away, and the state of meditation takes place.

To a purist, meditation is not a means to another end such as stress control. Zen practitioners would view seeking benefits from meditation as dualistic thinking. The experience is itself. You will value this if you meditate over an extended time. Although stress reduction is not the main point of meditation, it certainly is one of its powerful side effects.

There are many types and techniques of meditation to choose from. My favorite book on the topic is *Zen Mind, Beginner's Mind* (Weatherhill, 1970) by Shunryo Suzuki. Another helpful book is *Concentration and Meditation* by Christmas Humphreys (Shambhala, 1970).

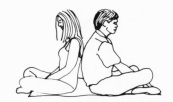

Couple Meditation

When you and your partner meditate together, a nonverbal bond gradually takes place which can expand your communication into areas often not explored together by couples. The experience is simply to meditate at your own pace in the same room as your partner is meditating. You may or may not want to talk about your experiences afterward.

Meditating while sitting back to back is also interesting. Each of you practices your meditation as you normally would but adds an awareness of your partner's breathing. Can you stay with your thoughts, feelings and breath patterns while also tuning in to your partner's body? Each time you become distracted and find yourself losing your own rhythm or arbitrarily synchronizing your breathing, relax and come back to your own breath rhythm. Can you feel your partner while maintaining your own rhythms? This will change at different times in your relationship.

Centering

Centering is the term for the basic idea of bringing your focus into your body to calm yourself. Controlling your breath pattern is the easiest and deepest method of controlling your tension level. The basic centering exercise involves relaxing your belly muscles and allowing the breath to sink deep into your abdomen. Your belly will rise as you inhale and sink as you exhale. Placing your hand across your abdomen just below your navel helps lower your breathing.

Focus your attention deep inside the center of your pelvis. The spiritual disciplines of the Orient view this area as the spiritual center, home base. Anytime you feel overrun by stress, focus your attention and breathing on your center and you will feel calmer.Centering in response to stress can become a reflex. Can you keep your focus and center of balance in your belly as you move, work, love?

Always have an ace in the hole.
                        Ella Fitzgerald

Aikido Centering Exercises

Aikido is a Japanese practice of self-defense and centering. Morihei Uyeshiba, a master of many Oriental forms of self-defense, developed Aikido late in his life while living in the mountains, studying the movements of birds and animals and meditating on the nature of self-defense.

The basic philosophy of Aikido is that to attack someone is to break the laws of the universe. It is to generate negative energy which will eventually come back against oneself. Who wins a conflict should not be determined by who has the biggest muscles or fancier weapons, but by who is more in tune with the universal spirit. The Japanese call this other power "Ki" or spirit. The Ki is dealt with as an actual molecular substance, an energy which moves and can be channeled and focused or "centered" in different parts of the body. It is the same as the "Chi" in Tai Chi Chuan. When the Ki is centered, a person is in a state of sensitivity, health, clarity and power. Many Aikido exercises will train you to be sensitive to the flow of your and another person's energy. If you are tuned in to an opponent's ki, know where he or she will move before he does and you will make sure you are not there. If you are attuned to a loved one's Ki, your emotional and physical interactions will be more like a dance.

I use some basic Aikido centering exercises, which I learned from Robert Nadeau in San Francisco, for relaxation and focus. Some are for centering your energy in your *hara*, or belly center, and others are for experimenting with centering in another body part and feeling how differently you can function with that focus change. Centering is directly related to good health. You can use centering exercises for self-healing. You can use centering exercises for stress reduction and for preparation for giving a massage.

The Mountain

Sit down comfortably cross-legged. Visualize a mountain and how it makes you feel. Now imagine that you are the mountain and that you feel as a mountain feels. What would you feel like if you had the qualities of a mountain: unmoving, massive and connected with the earth? Can you sit on the ground as a mountain rests without strain? There is comparatively little weight in the upper part of your body; the lower part of you is larger and heavier and anchors you to the ground. Stay with these mountain feelings and slowly stand up. Let your weight be evenly distributed on both feet and sink toward the ground through your legs. Experiment with walking as a mountain, very drawn to the earth, steady and powerful. Nothing distracts you from your centeredness or gets in your way. You are aware of yourself from your core to your exterior. How is this different from the way you usually sit and move? How could you use this exercise when you are feeling weak and scattered?

The Light Bulb

Imagine a light bulb in your lower abdomen. Turn it on and feel the little bit of heat the light gives inside you. How would it feel if you could breathe into this light bulb and with each breath make it a little brighter and warmer?

Imagine that you can allow this light and warmth to radiate out from your center and flow to all parts of your body, making each part glow and grow warm as the light moves through.

What would it feel like if you could project some of this light from the bulb in your center out of your body through your abdomen and into the air in front of you in a steady stream? Let the beam take on whatever qualities you need. Let it flow in any direction inside or outside your body as you wish. Do you want your energy now to be fast and concentrated, or slower and broader? Can you walk forward and let yourself move with this energy beam so that you feel the energy flowing through you and you flowing with it?

The Centered Brain

What would it be like if you had a second brain which rested in your abdomen, which could send messages out from your center? Imagine that this brain in your abdomen has been asleep and is now slowly waking up. It is becoming more aware of itself and aware of things around it. It is gradually awakening and wants to make a quiet sound as it stretches and opens up. What kind of sound would your abdomen brain make? Can you make the sound and let it come from deep in your center?

Let the sound gradually quiet down again. What would it feel like if the messages for your actions came from your center? Let yourself stand a moment with your eyes closed and your focus on that abdominal brain. What kind of movement would your new brain like to tell your body to make? Try to let the message come not from your usual head center, but from your lower abdomen feelings. Let yourself come to motion in this new way with the energy for action originating

67

in your center and flowing out to your different body parts for movement. Does this process feel different to you in any way from how you normally move? Experiment with simple actions like walking and imagine the energy for that movement coming from deep in your abdomen and spreading out into your legs and feet. The brain in your abdomen has different qualities from your head brain and with practice can open up new feelings and powers.

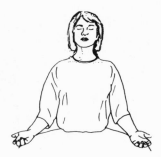

Self-Healing

Meditation and centering are two basic forms of self-healing because they are means of rearranging unbalanced energy (unhealth) and balancing (health) the flow throughout your body. Another approach is to use images. If you have an ear infection or a liver problem, for example, you could find a picture of a healthy ear or liver in a medical book and spend ten minutes a day visualizing your ear or liver to look like these healthy ones. You can also do the visual healing with someone else's ear or liver.

The basic idea is that the organ is "sick" because you have withdrawn the life energy from that part by tension. By focusing enough attention on the neglected parts and allowing life energy, spirit, and joy to move through them again, you can heal.

Healing Hands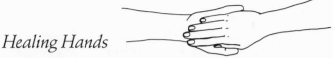

To prepare your hands use the palm centering exercise described in the *Fundamental Things to Apply* chapter. You can channel this healing energy throughout your body. It seems to be particularly strong through your arms and hands. To experiment simply place your right hand (palms down) on any spot on your partner's body which is tense and sore. Place your left palm on any other part of their body. (One especially good position is to have your hands opposite each other—that is your right hand, say, for stomach pain, on the stomach and your left hand opposite it on the back.) Close your eyes and relax your body. Center yourself and begin "exhaling" out your palms. You can also try imagining that the tension is moving from your right hand toward your left and dissipating. After five minutes or so, slowly take your hands away and ask your partner if any of the soreness or tension has gone.

Cow Cat

This exercise releases cramps and increases flexibility in your whole spine and pelvis. The lower back is the "joint" of the "upper and lower halves" of your body. Often movement is segmented here so that while a person moves her legs, for example in walking or running, she may hold her upper body rigid, or when she gestures using her arms and head, she may unconsciously hold the lower half of her body still. These tension producing habits can be changed by movements which allow your body to move smoothly as a whole. This exercise is particularly effective for releasing lower back tension.

On your hands and knees, inhale as you look up at the ceiling, and let your lower back sink down toward the floor as you arch your pelvis upward. This position is the "cow."

The "cat" is done as you exhale, curling your head and neck forward and tucking your pelvis under. Arch your middle back up toward the ceiling like a Halloween cat. Alternate these positions with your breathing, making the movements smooth and continuous.

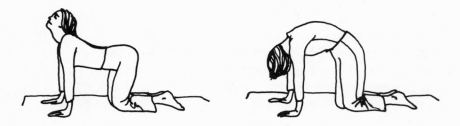

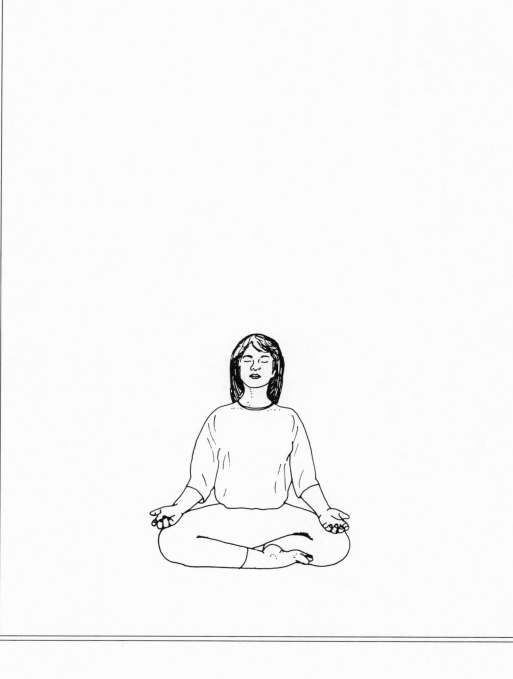

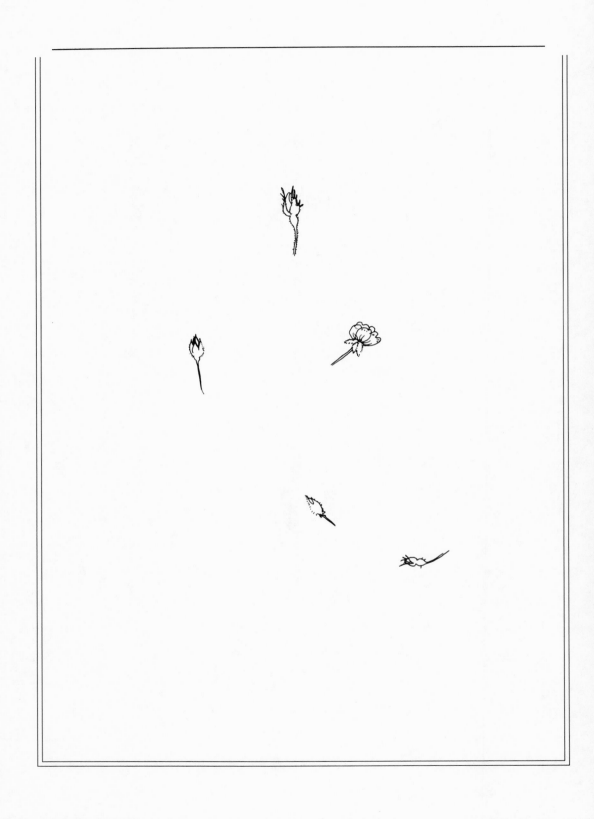

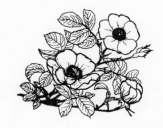

Picnic Massage

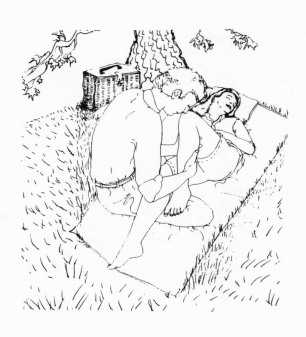

Picnic Massage

Back to Nature

For a friend who loves fresh air and green open spaces, a picnic plus massage can be the perfect special outing. Choose a place with a flat area where you can recline comfortably and one that is secluded enough that you won't be interrupted. A spectacular landscape increases the romantic sense of being transported to a magic realm.

A foot massage is an especially pleasant picnic treat. If you've been walking some distance, your lover will appreciate the pick-me-up. Clay based powders are a useful massage lubricant that won't be sticky when the relaxed feet return to their shoes. Herbal foot creams often contain wintergreen which stimulates circulation, and the creams are easily absorbed. The Body Shop's *Peppermint Foot Lotion* is terrific.

Eating lunch after the massage is the most comfortable. Stay in partial shade so that your friend does not become too hot during the massage. Place a pillow under the head and knees and bring one for you to sit comfortably. Be thorough in your massage, but twenty minutes is about as long as you can go if you want the receiver to stay awake to enjoy the picnic and the hike.

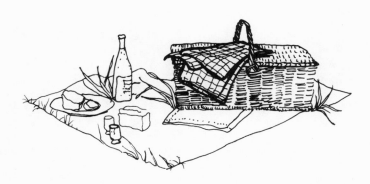

A Picnic Foot Massage

15 minutes

Ankle Circles

Overlapping Squeezes

Arch Fist

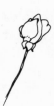

Metatarsal Folds

Side Pinches

Tendon Valleys

Toe Twirls

Tendon Fans

Overlapping Squeezes

Palm Rests

A Picnic Foot Massage

Ankle Circles

Thoroughly massage one foot, then the other.
Rest the foot in your lap or on a pillow.
Lightly oil or powder the ankle of one foot.
Using the fingertips of both hands, make firm,
slow circles around the ankle bones.

Now move just above the ankle bones and circle the ankle
with your fingers. With your thumbs facing each other on
top and your fingers facing each other from underneath, clasp
one ankle with both hands. Alternate rotating your hands
away from each other around the ankle and then toward each
other in a firm, wringing motion. With sufficient oil, this
stroke feels great.

Overlapping Squeezes

Pick up the right foot with both hands.
Your thumbs will be on top of the foot just
below the ankle and your fingers will be on
the sole. Move your hands in an overlapping, squeezing motion. Drag one hand
toward the toes. Before this hand leaves the
foot, start the squeeze motion with your
other hand. Squeeze hard and speed up.
Then gradually slow the pace again.

Arch Fist

Steady the top of the foot with your left
hand. With the knuckles of your hands in a
fist, massage the sole. Move in small circles
and press hard.

Metatarsal Folds

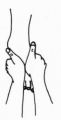

With the heels of both hands against the top of the foot and your fingertips pressing into the middle of the sole, press very hard down onto the top of the foot and up into the sole. At the same time, slowly slide the heels of your hands from the middle of the foot out to the edges. Repeat this several times.

Side Pinches

Squeeze the outer edge of the foot between your thumb and fingers. Move methodically along the outer edge from the little toe to the far tip of the heel.

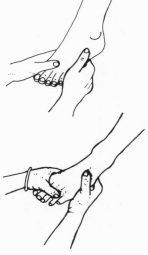

Tendon Valleys

On the top of the foot find the long tendons running from the base of the ankle to each toe. Slide the tip of your thumb all the way down each of the valleys between the tendons. Hard pressure feels good here.

Toe Twirls

With your left hand steady the foot. With the thumb and forefinger of your right hand grasp the base of the big toe. Firmly pull and twist in a corkscrew motion, until your thumb and forefinger slide off the end of the toe. Do each toe carefully.

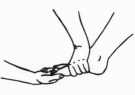

Tendon Fans

Using a hand on each foot, grasp both feet with your fingers on the soles and the heels of your hands on the top of the feet. You are gripping each foot just above the little toes. Squeeze as you slide the heels of your hands from the center of the foot out toward the little toes. Your hands will trace a crescent path as they slide off the feet. Move to the spots where you started and squeeze both feet again.

Overlapping Squeezes

Repeat the squeeze down the arch but this time vary it by using one hand on each foot. With both hands pull down on the feet so your thumbs massage the top of the feet and your fingers press into the arches. Repeat several times.

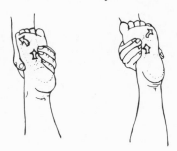

Palm Rests

Sandwich a foot between your hands, one palm resting on the sole and one on the top. For a moment rest there. Center and become aware of your breathing. Imagine that you're sending your breath through your hands to reach the energy in your partner's foot. Repeat on the other foot.

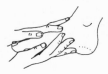

This massage will make your love feel younger than Springtime!

Reflexology Massage

Reflexology is based on the idea that there are nerves and electromagnetic energy pathways from all parts of the body connecting with the feet. By pressing quite firmly on the spot on your foot which corresponds to your problem area, you can have a positive influence on an ailment, improving circulation to that organ and stimulating energy and nerve connections.

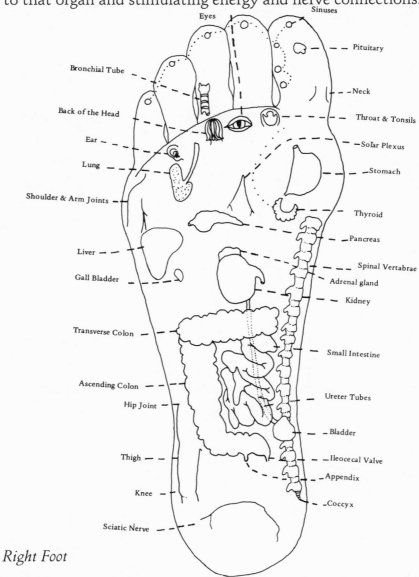

Eyes
Sinuses
Pituitary
Bronchial Tube
Neck
Back of the Head
Throat & Tonsils
Ear
Solar Plexus
Lung
Stomach
Shoulder & Arm Joints
Thyroid
Pancreas
Liver
Spinal Vertabrae
Gall Bladder
Adrenal gland
Kidney
Transverse Colon
Small Intestine
Ascending Colon
Ureter Tubes
Hip Joint
Bladder
Thigh
Ileocecal Valve
Appendix
Knee
Coccyx
Sciatic Nerve

Right Foot

Some pressure points will feel neutral or good; some may be sore. With continued massage, the area should relax and feel better. You can stimulate reflexology points as you do your picnic massage.

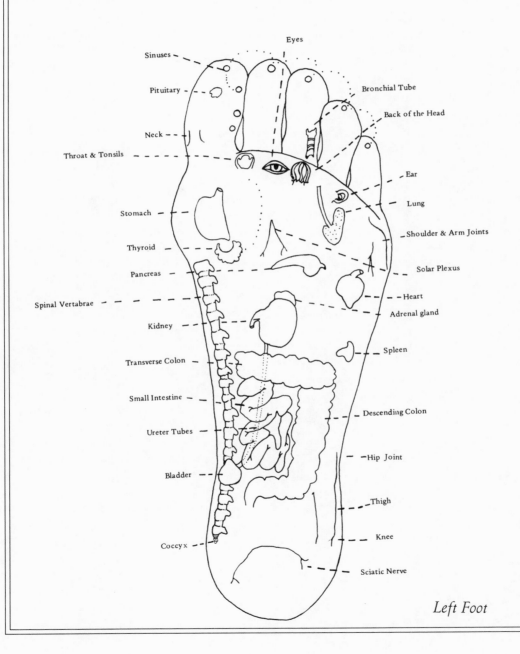

Left Foot

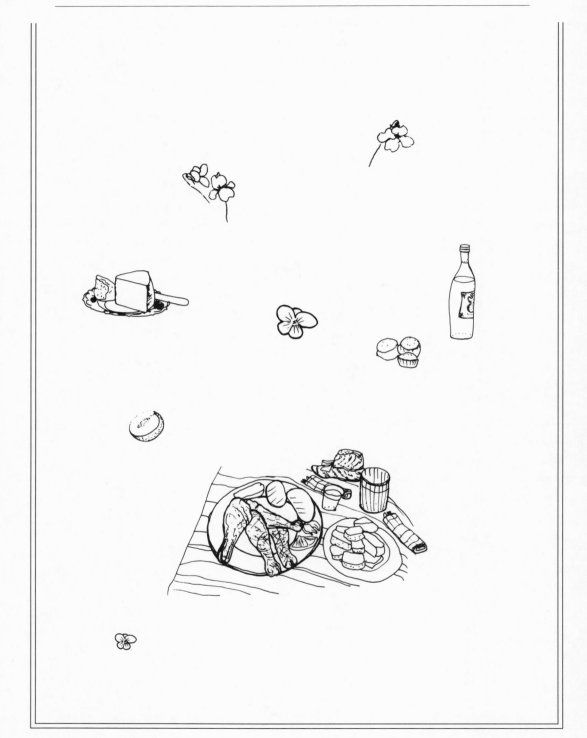

Country Picnic

Cold Roast Chicken

Marinated Asparagus

Bread and Saga Blue Cheese

Limeade or White Wine in Thermos

Kendall's Mint Cake

Fresh Peaches and Blueberries

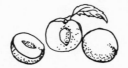

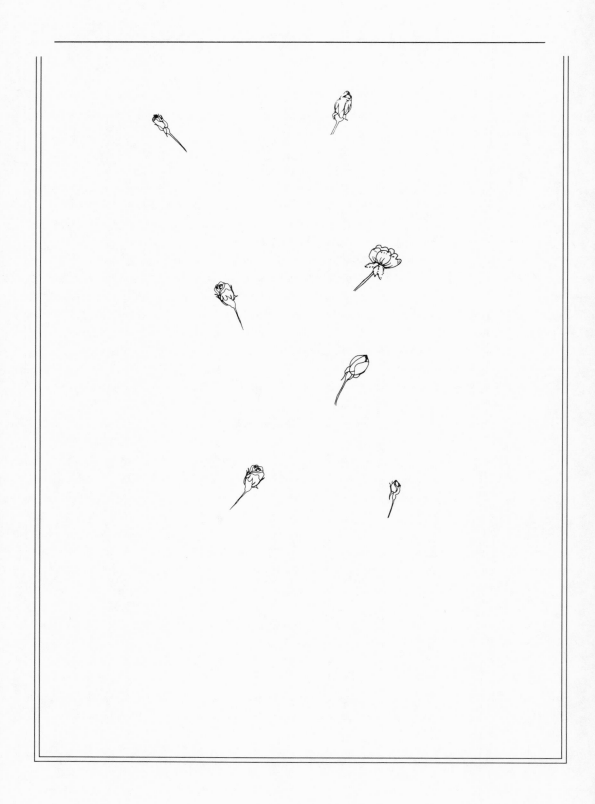

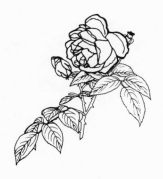

Sweet Dreams Massage

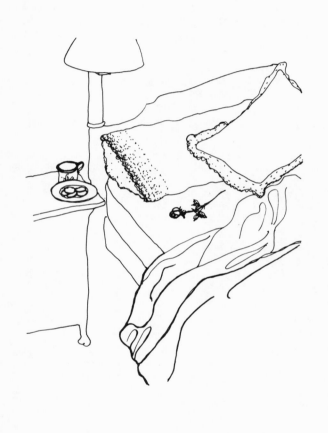

Sweet Dreams Massage

Want your lover to have sweet dreams of you? Put him or her to bed with a soothing massage.

There are moments when the most wonderful gift you can give your lover is the gift of sleep. You can share a hot drink, talk over the day, and then ease any tensions with a massage.

On Hands

Hand massage is a particularly pleasant goodnight. Hands are the physical resting places of many of our compulsive tensions because our hands are the vehicles for most of our work actions and chores. Quieting the hands releases surprising amounts of stress. Special attention to the palms and fingers feels intimate because of the great number of nerve endings on the inside of the hand. Stroking and holding the hands conveys a deep sense of security that is reassuring at night and conducive to sleep. Attention to hands is a courtly form of homage and a classical expression of devotion to a lover.

Goodnight, sweet prince or princess.

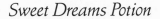

Sweet Dreams Potion

Serve before the massage to help your love fall asleep.

Hot milk with almond extract, honey and cinnamon sprinkle

 or Hot Toddy

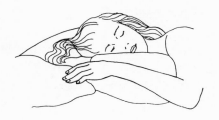

Sweet Dreams Hand Massage
15 Minutes

Palm Sandwich

Palm Folds

Palm Fist

Finger Twirls

Forearm Slides

Palm Sandwich

Feathers

Palm Sandwich

Hold your lover's hand lightly sandwiched between both of yours, contacting as much of its surface as you can. Close your eyes and focus on your own breathing. Then focus on your friend's hand and imagine you can send the energy from your hands into your lover's.

Palm Folds

Lightly oil the hands. Hold the palm gently in both your hands. Then press the heels of your hand against the middle of the back of the hand and press the tips of your fingers into the middle of the palm. Now press hard upward with your fingertips and downward with the heels of your hands from the 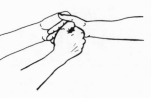 middle of the hand to the edges. Move the heels of your hands together again and repeat the motion. The opposing pressure allows you to squeeze and fold the hand and to "drain" any tension.

Palm Fist

Place your lover's hand in the palm of your hand. Make a fist with your other hand and massage the palm in firm circles with your knuckles. Repeat on the other palm. Try to massage in between the bones of the hand.

Finger Twirls

Rest your lover's hand in your left hand. With your thumb and forefinger lightly grasp the base of the thumb. Pull your thumb and fore- 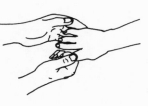 finger firmly from base to top of the thumb, twisting your hand in a spiral corkscrew motion around the thumb as you go. Slide off the tip. Do each finger in the same way.

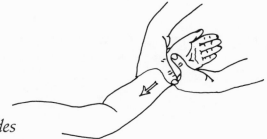

Forearm Slides

Spread some oil on your lover's forearm. Gently raise the forearm until it is upright with the elbow against the bed. Ring the wrist with the thumbs and forefingers of your hands. Both thumbs touch flat on the inside of the wrist. Now squeeze with your thumbs and forefingers and slide both hands down the forearm. Move slowly. At the crook of the elbow, slide your hands back up to the wrist, keeping your fingers in contact with the skin but not pressing. The pleasure of this stroke comes from the rhythmic pressing downward and releasing upward as you "drain" the arm.

Palm Sandwich

Repeat earlier stroke on other hand.

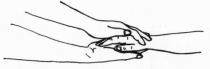

Feathers

With your fingertips make light strokes with overlapping hand motions down the forearm, over the hand and off the fingers. Let one feather stroke start before the other ends so the sensation is continuous. Use lighter and lighter pressure until you lift your hands away entirely and allow your love to sleep peacefully.

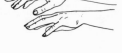

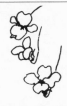

Dream Lovers

Herbs can be used to fill a Dream Pillow which is placed under your pillow to influence your dreams. Or you can make a dream sachet for your lover to keep under his or her pillow. Use somewhat porous material such as linen, silk or lace so the aroma is clear. Combine the ingredients according to your preferences. Lavender blossoms, coriander seeds, laurel, absinthe and roses all attract love. Add some mint leaves, cloves or violets to enlist happiness in love. Comfrey leaves and eucalyptus encourage good health. Hops encourage restful sleep. Artemesia herb encourages prophetic dreams. Dry the herbs. Fill the sachet. Sleep on it.

It is sometimes possible to decide your dreams before you go to sleep. Choose an event or question that concerns both you and your lover. Tell yourself to dream your deep feelings and best answers and to remember the dream in the morning. Often this self-instruction is effective and you'll wake up with new insights.

Sometimes people spontaneously participate in each other's dreams. Share your dreams with each other regularly. Telling dreams out loud also helps you to remember future dreams. Sweet dreams.

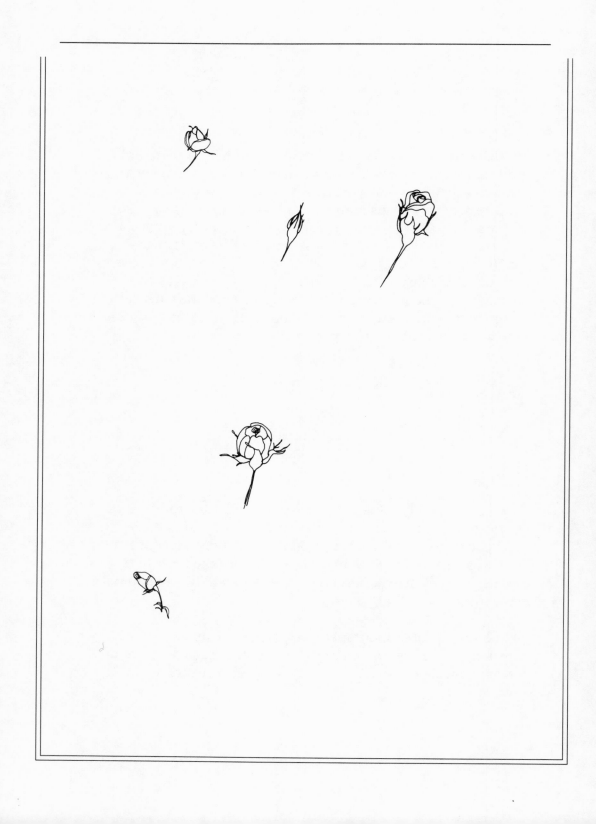

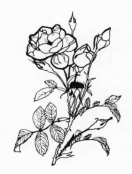

Happy New Year Massage

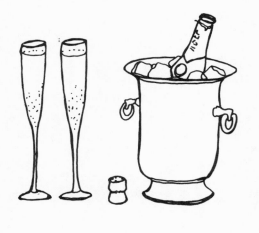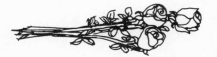

Happy New Year Massage

Start the New Year Relaxed and Right

When you want someone to say, "Our love is here to stay," start their year with a memorable massage.

New Year's Eve is often an evening of dancing. The following is a thorough leg massage that can be done several hours before your evening's events. When your love is ready to step out, he or she will be walking on air. Or you can give it on New Year's Day as an antidote to kicking up your heels the night before. Whichever time you choose, the leg massage will ensure that your love puts the best foot forward into the New Year.

Do, Do, Do What You Done, Done, Done Before

New Year's Eve is the traditional time to take stock of the old and plan for the new, a time to reminisce about shared experiences. Knowing your lover remembers something special you did makes you feel appreciated.

Unforgettable That's What You Are

You can write a Romantic Resolutions list of loving things you plan to do in the coming year and give it to your lover.

In the meantime, promise her anything, but give her a massage.

Happy New Year Massage

20 Minutes

If convenient, time this to end on the stroke of midnight.

Double Main Stroke

Thumbs on Calves

Draining the Calf

Back of Knee Circles

Thigh Slides

Thigh Waves

Knee Bend

Feet Squeezes

Feathers and Ripples

Double Main Stroke

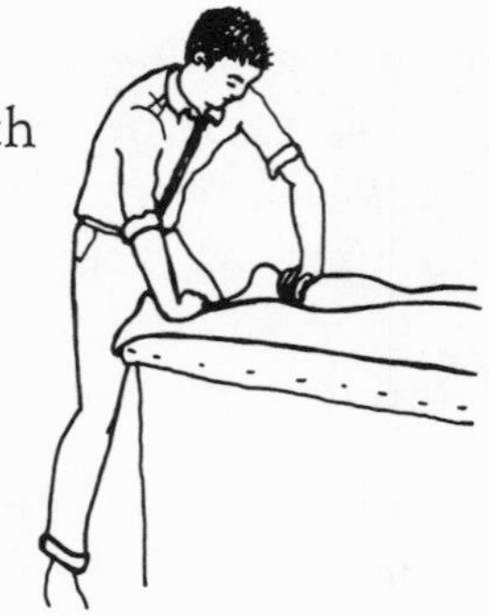

Your lover is lying on his or her stomach with the head to which ever side is comfortable. Spread oil on the legs, buttocks and hips.

Place the feet about a foot apart. Stand beside the left foot. Place your left hand across the ankle with your fingertips pointing toward the right and your right hand on the right ankle with fingertips pointing toward the left side of the table. Move both hands up the legs lightly over the back of the knee, but otherwise apply a lot of

96

pressure by leaning down. As you move your arms up the legs you'll need to walk forward beside the bed or table. At the top of the thigh glide your hands over the buttocks until the fingertips locate the hip bones. Slide the hands down the hip to the bed, tracing the curve of the bones. Then pull your hands down both legs to the ankles. When your hands near the ankle, pivot them to your starting position without breaking the flow of your movement.

Repeat this stroke several times. You can return to it at different points during a massage whenever you want to impart a sense of wholeness to the massage.

Thumbs on Calves

Now use the balls of your thumbs to massage the calf muscles. Slide your thumbs away from you in short, alternating strokes with deep pressure over the back of the foreleg. Keep the strokes continuous for the best sensation.

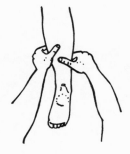

Draining the Calf

Your palms cup either side of the leg at the ankle, your fingers pointing toward the bed. Both thumbs cross the base of the calf pointing in toward each other and lying side by side.

Slide your hands up the leg squeezing your palms and thumbs. Just before you reach the knee slowly and with no pressure, slide your hands down the foreleg. The thumbs stay side by side, throughout the stroke. Go up and back several times, applying pressure during the upward movement only.

Back of Knee Circles

With the fingers of one hand trace light circles in the hollow area in back of the knee. To feel best the stroke should be feathery.

Thigh Slides

Leaning on the heels of your hands, slide in overlapping strokes. Start the second stroke just before ending the first so the sensation is continuous. Work at first in short slides and then longer ones covering more leg area. You can continue the slide up onto hips and buttocks.

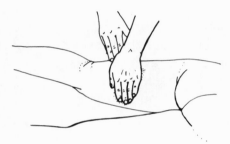

Thigh Waves

On the inside of the thigh just above the knee, draw your hands upward in very slow alternating strokes. Keeping the palms touching the skin and the fingers pointing toward the bed, start a new stroke as you are finishing the previous one. The pressure is gentle, and the rhythm should be slow and steady.

Start each stroke a little higher up the leg until you come to the pelvis. Then work back down toward the knee.

Knee Bend

You can lift the foreleg and bend it back toward the buttock up to the point at which the foreleg resists being pushed back. Push the heel of the foot toward the buttock and allow a few more inches if you can do it without straining. Next lower the leg back to the table.

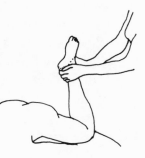

Feet Squeezes

Use some extra oil on the feet for this stroke. Pick up the left foot with both your hands. Have your thumbs on the sole of the foot and the rest of your fingers on the top. Move your hands in an overlapping, squeezing motion. Start with your left thumb at the base of the heel. Squeeze the foot with your left hand and drag your hand down the foot to the base of the toes. Press hard with your thumb. Just before your left thumb reaches the base of the toes, begin the same squeezing and dragging with your right thumb. Now pick up your left hand and start the stroke over at the base of the heel.

Try it at different speeds. You can also massage both feet at once by using one hand per foot and squeezing and pulling downward simultaneously.

Feathers and Ripples

This is a pleasant stroke almost anywhere. It works well on the back of the leg, the buttocks, the hips and back. Hold both hands with your fingers stiff and spread apart and slightly curved. Drag your fingers lightly down the length of the leg with alternating strokes. Begin at the top of the leg or, if you want, on the buttock itself.

Go down the whole of both legs. This stroke usually feels best when done in the downward direction; however, some people enjoy the other direction also. You can vary it by tracing wavy lines with your fingers. Your pressure should become lighter and lighter until you raise your hands off the body.

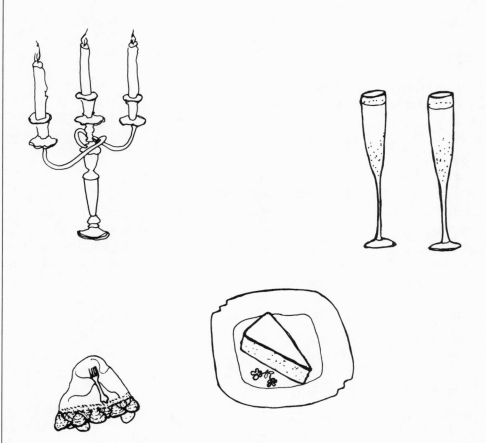

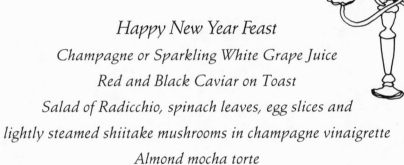

Happy New Year Feast
Champagne or Sparkling White Grape Juice
Red and Black Caviar on Toast
Salad of Radicchio, spinach leaves, egg slices and
lightly steamed shiitake mushrooms in champagne vinaigrette
Almond mocha torte

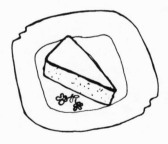

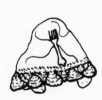

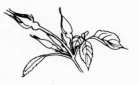

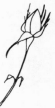

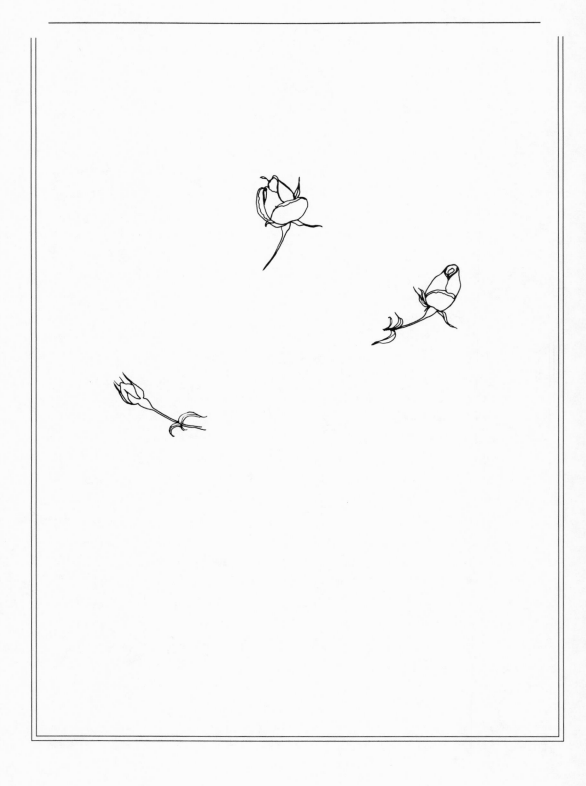

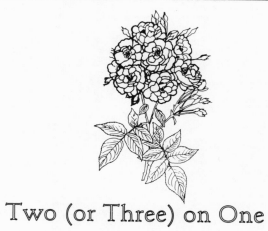

Two (or Three) on One

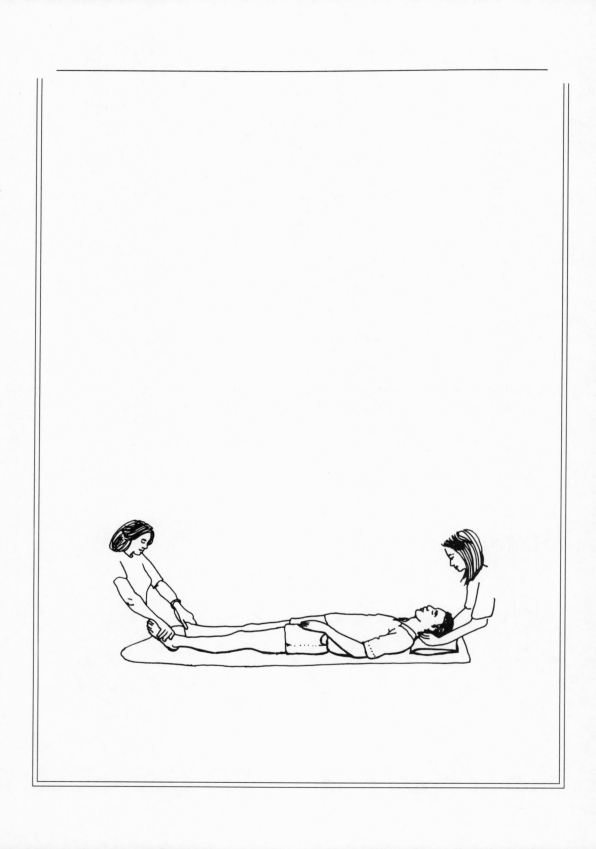

Two (or Three) on One

The More the Merrier

It takes two to tango, but sometimes it takes three to give an unforgettable massage. If your lover agrees with Mae West that too much is just enough, he or she will probably enjoy a multiple person massage. It's fun for everyone, and there are some techniques you can do with two people massaging that one person can't do. There's even a school of two-masseur massage developing called Quatre Mains, meaning four hands in French.

If you are giving the massage, working with another person is stimulating because their actions inspire you to do new movements and invent new strokes. For the person receiving the massage, the experience is a luxury. If it's great to have one person taking care of you, imagine how divine it is to have two or even three people taking care of you.

The people massaging need to combine their strokes so that they are coordinated and not chaotic. Then a quatre mains massage can be a great pleasure.

Nothing Succeeds Like Excess

A powerful feeling of integration results from several parts of your body being massaged at once. You lose any sense of segments and feel a wonderful wholeness.

The cast of masseurs and masseuses can be several friends, or family, even children. The experience can also raise the pleasure quotas of the givers. It is satisfying to work and play together to care for someone you love.

Two (or Three) on One

One Half Hour

Double Breath Centering

Scalp and Feet Rubs

Double Main Stroke

Double Palm Slides

Backs of Knees and Elbows Circles

Feathers on Arms

Shoulder Rotations

Hip Rotations

Double Thigh Waves

Palm and Sole Circles

Feather Sweeps

Two (or Three) on One

Massaging with partners is a natural time for inventing strokes because other people's movements as well as the restrictions of this type of massage inspire new techniques. Certain strokes lend themselves most easily to two-person massaging. These appear in the following massage. The directions describe two people doing the massage, however, three or more could easily join without creating chaos by coordinating with the others. For example, a lucky receiver could possibly have a masseur on each hand and each foot.

Put your children to work. Then trade and give them the multiple treat.

Double Breath Centering

If two people are massaging one, each of you sits or stands at an opposite end of your friend's body. One places his or her palms on each foot. The other rests palms on the head. Remain still several moments with your eyes closed and relax your breathing. Imagine you can exhale warmth through your arms and hands. When you feel relaxed begin the strokes.

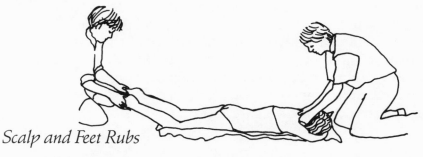

Scalp and Feet Rubs

Curl the fingers of both hands and rub the scalp on both sides of the head with your fingertips. Moving your left hand in small circles, press hard enough that the skin moves a bit over the bone. Cover the entire scalp with your circles.

Your friend is simultaneously using fingertips to massage the soles of the feet. Use deep pressure and be thorough. Keep the same pace in your strokes as your partner working on the head.

Double Main Stroke

The person at the feet glides both hands, fingers pointing in opposite directions and pressure on heels of hands, up the back of one leg. At the top of the leg, continue over the buttock and up one side of the back.

109

Now the person at the head goes to the outer shoulder and joins in the back massage. Both masseurs bring their hands heels first down the side of the back and then the legs, all the way back to the ankles, the stroke going up the body now with someone massaging each leg. Do this stroke up and down the body several times.

Double Palm Slides

Stand or sit on opposite sides of your friend's back. Each of you places your palms down on your side of the back. Glide your palms in horizontal strips across the back. Pull your right hand toward yourself as you push your left hand away from yourself, and vice versa. Keep the hands moving constantly, rapidly without leaving the surface of the skin. Stagger the placement of your four arms so that you slide between each other's hands. Starting at the shoulders work gradually down to the waist and back up again. Establish a steady coordinated rhythm so you are working as one.

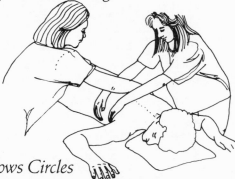

Backs of Knees and Elbows Circles

Use a circular stroking with your fingertips on the backs of the knees and elbows. Each of you circles one hand on the back of one knee while circling the other hand in the crook of the arm. Then circle the opposite elbow and knee areas. Since four hands are available try different combinations of circling in different areas at the same time.

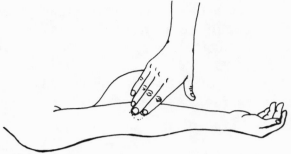

Feathers on Arms

From the palms, each masseur begins light, slow strokes with their fingertips up the arms, across the shoulders and onto the upper back. Now reverse the direction and angle your stroking down the arms again. These kinds of strokes keep your spot work connected to the rest of the body in a pleasant way. Experiment with feathery stroking connecting the arms to other parts of the body. Now the person turns over onto the back as you continue the feather stroking on the arms and shoulders.

Shoulder Rotations

Each masseur places one hand on a shoulder and the other under an elbow. Lift up each arm and draw a circle in the air with the shoulder. The person being massaged should relax and allow the two masseurs to do all the work of lifting the limbs. Giving over the movement to the masseurs allows the joints to release tension. When lifting, coordinate your pace and direction with your partner's.

Hip Rotations

Having one's limbs lifted gently allows deep relaxation for the person being massaged. Try the technique on the hip joints which are often tense. Each masseur stands beside a leg and slips his or her outside palm under one thigh while placing the hand closest to the massaged friend's body on top of the thigh or you can place one hand at the ankle. Lift the legs a few inches off the bed so that each masseur can make small, slow circles with the leg to rotate the hip. Then slowly lower the limbs down again. If you are being massaged, try to allow the two people to move your legs so your muscles will relax thoroughly. Being lifted this way can recall pleasant child-hood feelings of being securely carried.

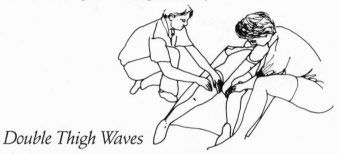

Double Thigh Waves

On the inside of the thigh just above the knee, draw your hands upward in slow, hand-over-hand strokes. Begin a new hand slide just as you are finishing the previous one. The pressure is gentle, the rhythm steady, and the palms stay in contact with the skin. Move up the leg as you go and continue the stroke on the other thigh. Try to coordinate your rhythm with the person's strokes on the opposite thigh. This overlapping stroke also feels wonderful on the sides of the torso and hips.

Palm and Sole Circles

Each masseur makes circles with the fingertips in the palm of one hand and the arch of one foot.

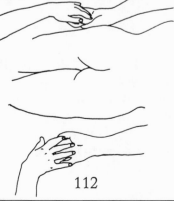

Feather Sweeps

Using very light fingertip pressure, the masseurs glide their hands across both palms, down the length of the fingers, and off the fingertips. After repeating this stroking motion several times, the extra masseur can quietly exit to leave the two lovers alone together as the remaining masseur continues the light feathery stroking all over the back of the body.

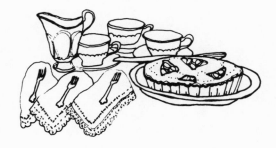

Tea for Three

Hot Earl Grey Tea in Thermos

Cream, sugar, lemon

Cucumber, parsley and butter sandwiches

Apricot tart

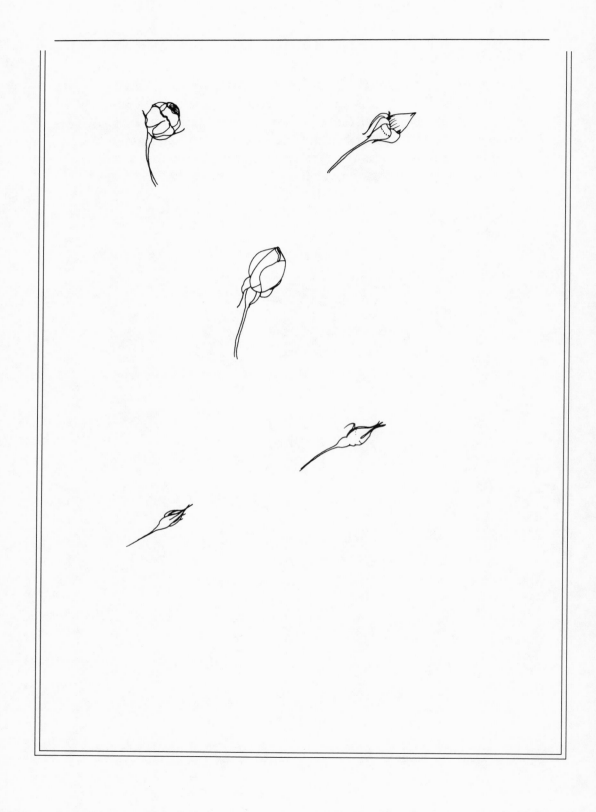

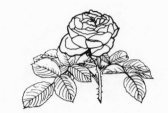

Be My Valentine

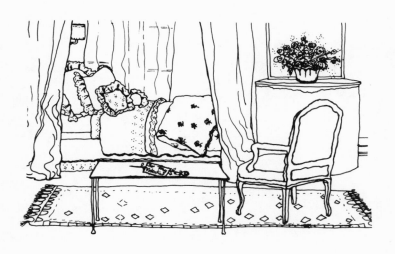

Be My Valentine

Whether you can afford daily champagne and caviar, or you can't give anything but love, the most romantic gift you can offer is the gift of yourself. Key ingredients are still a kiss, a sigh and a loving touch. Here's a massage your lover will love.

Massage for Lovers

One Hour or More

♡ *Marks the Half Hour Short but Sweet Variation*

♡ Long Feathers
♡ Feet Treats
Fingernail Feathers
♡ Palm Waves
♡ Kisses
♡ Thigh Waves
♡ Waterfall
Cupid's Arrow
♡ Kneading Buttocks
Shoulder Circles
Scalp Rub
♡ Main Stroke on Chest and Stomach
Belly Circles
Breast Figure Eight
♡ Nipple Stars
Navel Spirals
♡ Thigh Waves
Double Knee Circles
Palm Folds
Five Finger Palm Rub
♡ Arch Circles
Lovers' Knots
♡ Full Feathers

You Do Something to Me That Nobody Else Can Do

This massage can be as sensual for the giver as for the receiver. Previous boundaries can be laid aside, and anything goes. Both giver and receiver are nude to enhance the eroticism of the exchange. Improvisation in lovers' massage is open to techniques such as licking, scratching lightly, tickling, heated towels or breathing to warm body parts and any other inventions you both enjoy.

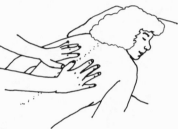

♡ *Long Feathers*

Your lover can start lying on his or her stomach so you can massage the back first. Place your palms on your lover's shoulders. Draw them along the muscles on either side of the spine down the back and over the hips down the legs. As you cross the arches, angle your hands away from each other and lift them off the body. Make this a continuous, overlapping, sweeping motion. Return your palms to the shoulders and begin the sweep again with light strokes that are slow and gradually speed up. Try the same stroking with only one index finger and very slowly trace the contours of your lover's back, hips, legs and feet. Start on the face and work slowly down to the toes. Trace in between the toes and around the heels and ankles. Activities such as dancing and romancing all night can put extra strain on the hip joints so don't neglect the area. This can also be a highly sensual area for certain people.

♡ *Feet Treats*

Because feet are so sensitive, many people experience erotic pleasure from gentle, slow foot massage. On well oiled feet, slide one finger between each pair of toes in a spiral motion going in and straight coming out.

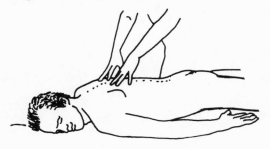

Fingernail Feathers

As Oscar Wilde observed, "Simple pleasures are the last refuge of the complex." Some of the most sophisticated people I know prefer the simplest of massages: light fingernail scratching all over the body.

When the scratching is done extremely lightly, it *almost* tickles and is usually experienced as erotically exciting. However, when the stroking is done with medium pressure, the effect is very soothing. Remember the crocodile tamer's technique? Use all your fingers, and experiment with different circular, fan, overlapping, spiral and straight patterns of stroking.

♡ *Palm Waves*

Now oil the back of your lover with long overlapping strokes of your palms. Have a squeeze bottle of massage oil within reach or a bowl. Keep some part of your arm or body touching your lover when you reach for more oil. You want to maintain continuous physical touch throughout the massage. Begin spreading oil on the soles of the feet.

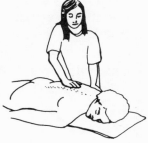

Then cover the backs of the legs in overlapping upward strokes. Cover the buttocks, back, arms and hands.

Once the body is oiled, deep pressure feels good. With the heels of your hands press firmly and glide your hands up the arms until they meet on the upper back. Continue down the back, over the hips and onto the backs of the thighs.

♡ Kisses

The kiss, like carbon, is one of the basic elements of life. Kissing is an unbeatable romantic massage element. I'm sure you can think of delightful places for kisses and sprinkle them throughout your massage.

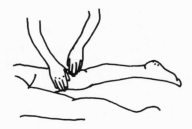

♡ Thigh Waves

The inner thigh area is especially sensitive to delicate touch and often a favorite erotic massage zone.

On the inside of the thigh just above the knee, draw your hands upward in slow, hand-over-hand strokes. Begin a new hand slide just as you are finishing the previous one. The pressure is gentle, the rhythm is steady, and the palms stay in contact with the skin. Move up the leg as you go, to the crease between the leg and the buttock. You can continue this gentle overlapping stroke across the buttocks and hips. Then stroke the other thigh in the same pattern.

♡ *Waterfall*

After you have completed the wave stroke on both thighs, move to the tailbone and place your right palm on the sacrum, fingers pointing toward you. Slide your two hands as a unit up the spine, keeping a steady, moderate pressure. (Never press down hard directly on the spine.) At the top of the spine, reverse the motion with the tips of the first two fingers of your right hand pressing into the muscles on either side of the vertebrae. Slide your fingertips two or three inches down the muscles on either side of the spine. Then begin the same pressing, sliding motion with the first two fingertips of your left hand, covering the area your right hand has just covered. Lift your right hand and slide the fingers of your left hand an inch or so farther down the back.

Keep repeating this alternating sliding and pressing with your fingertips on both sides of the spine. As one pair of fingertips is pressing, raise the other off the back. Then start the motion with your other hand.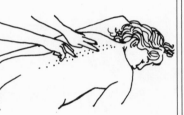

On the receiving end the stroke correctly done will feel like a waterfall or having something smooth roll down the back.

Cupid's Arrow

Bring your hands to the lower spine. The sacrum is a flat bone at the base of the spine, shaped like an arrowhead pointing to the feet. With your fingertips, press and trace the

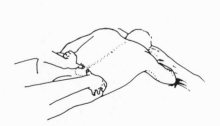
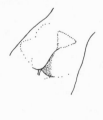

outline of the sacrum by moving them away from either side of the spine at the top of the sacrum, to the tips, and down the sides to the tailbone. When you reach the tip reverse the motion and slide your fingertips back up the sides and across the top, until they come together again on either side of the spine. You can add several overlapping thumb strokes on top of the arrow bone as you finish.

♡ Kneading Buttocks

Knead the flesh of either buttock as if you were preparing bread dough. Lift and squeeze the flesh between the thumb and your fingers rhythmically, alternating hands. Knead one buttock thoroughly and then the other. Continue this stroke onto the muscles of the back.

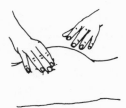

Shoulder Circles

Move to a comfortable position behind your partner's head. Make firm circles with the heels of your hands on the long shoulder muscles to either side of the neck. Now with the fingertips and nails of one hand make very light slow circles on the back of the neck where it moves into the shoulders.

Now is the time to ask your partner to roll slowly over onto the back.

Scalp Rub

With the pads of your fingers, use both hands to make small circles all over the scalp. To reach the back of the skull, lift and turn the head slightly to one side. Supporting the head with one palm, massage with the other hand. Then repeat the massage on the other side of the scalp. Tension causes the thin muscle layer covering the scalp to tighten.

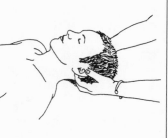

Massaging the scalp improves hair condition and alleviates headaches and nervous tension. Most people find scalp massage relaxing and comforting.

Many people find the mastoid bone of the scalp very sensual so concentrate some massage there. The mastoid bones are semi-circular and curved behind the ear. Use the fingertips of both hands to massage in crescent arcs along the back of the ear. Draw your hands from the bed up toward the temples. Include some light circles on the neck, the temples and the forehead.

♡ Main Stroke on Chest and Stomach

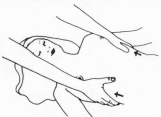

Sit or stand above your friend's head. Place both palms on the middle of the chest with the heels of your hands just below the collarbone. Your fingers point toward teach other. Now slide your hands forward, pressing firmly on the chest and more lightly on the stomach. When your hands reach the lower stomach, with your fingers pointing toward the feet, spread both hands out to the sides. Now slide your hands down the hips all the way to the bed. Then begin to pull them along the sides of the torso up toward the shoulders. Pull firmly as if you were about to draw your lover a few inches down the bed.

As you reach the armpits pull your hands, heels first, up onto the top of the chest. Pivot each hand on its heel, the fingertips face the center of the chest. Glide from here into more of the same stroke.

Belly Circles

The person being massaged should have the knees bent while you are massaging the stomach. You can place the legs in the right position or you can raise the legs and put a pillow under them. Sit or stand at your lover's right side and begin slow wide circles on the stomach with the palm of your left hand, moving clockwise because the colon coils clockwise. Circle just below the ribs, then a bit onto the right side of the torso at the waist, then just above the pelvic bone, then a bit onto the right side of the torso at the waist.

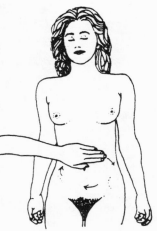

After a complete circle add the right hand to make a half circle. After the left hand has passed from the lower to the upper half of the stomach, the right hand smooths half of a circle from hip to hip along the pelvic bone. When the right hand reaches the right hip, raise it in the air over the left hip so that it can repeat the same crescent movement after the left hand has completed another circle. Whenever the right hand is massaging, it should be opposite the left hand.

Breast Figure Eight

This stroke is designed for a woman, but it feels equally pleasant on a man's chest. Your friend is lying down on her back. Sit on her right side about parallel to her waist, so that your left arm can easily reach her chest. Spread oil all over your friend's torso.

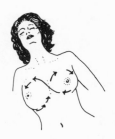

124

The pattern of this stoke is a figure eight on the muscles supporting the breasts. Your right hand should be resting *lightly* on your partner's abdomen. Use your left palm and fingers to describe the figure eight. Begin on the sternum bone in between her breasts, your fingers pointing away from you. Lean some of your weight onto your left palm and slide it around the lower edge of your friend's left breast. Move around her side, and up onto the pectoral muscles. Now move your hand, heel first, down under your friend's right breast, up her right side, and back onto the upper chest by way of her pectoral muscle—until you end up touching the place on the sternum where you began the stoke. Keep circling continuously around the breasts in this figure eight several times.

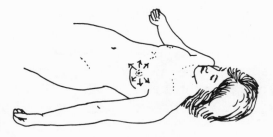

♡ Nipple Stars

This stroke feels delightful on a man or a woman. Position your thumbs on either side of the nipple. With light pressure slide your thumbs apart to reach the edges of the breast, or about five inches apart on a man. Pick up your thumbs and return them to the center to repeat the spreading motion in spokes around the nipple. Repeat on the other breast.

Navel Spirals

The star stoke feels good around the navel also.

For another intriguing navel stroke, use your forefingers, begin at the navel and draw larger and larger circles around it. Spiral out with the navel as the center until you are describing circles bordered by the ribs and the pelvic bones.

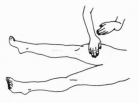

♡ Thigh Waves

On the inside of the thigh just above the knee, draw your hands upward in slow, hand-over-hand stokes. Begin a new hand slide just as you are finishing the previous one. The pressure is gentle, the rhythm steady, and the palms stay in contact with the skin. Move up the leg as you go and continue the stroke on the other thigh. This overlapping stroke also feels wonderful on the sides of the torso and hips.

Double Knee Circles

Knees, prime targets of sports and tension injuries, deserve careful massage. Knees are also an area of sensual pleasure exciting enough to some Frenchmen to name romantic films after them, so try some special attention there to find out how your lover feels about knees. Sitting beside the knees, use both your thumbs to outline circles around the kneecaps. Brace your fingers, like a post of a draughtsman's compass and describe slow circles using both thumbs at once. Then make smooth circles using all your fingers on the outside, then the inside, then the back of each knee. Now glide both palms using firm pressure up the legs, over the hips, across the chest and onto the shoulders. Bring each palm down the arms to begin massage on the hands.

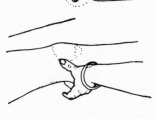

Palm Folds

Hold your lover's hand in both your hands. The heels of your hands press against the

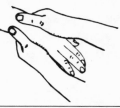

126

back of the hand. Your fingertips press against the middle of the palm underneath. The heels of your hands touch each other. Now press hard upward with your fingertips and downward with the heels of your hands. Simultaneously, slowly slide the heels of your hands out to the edges where you stop. Do this squeezing motion several times. Slow and hard feels great.

Five Finger Palm Rub

Want to discover a different position? Try this one. Hold your lover's hand in a new way. With your lover's palm up, place the little finger of your left hand between the forefinger and middle finger; the fourth and middle finger of your left hand between the forefinger and thumb; and the forefinger of your left hand on the other side of the thumb. At the same time place the little finger of your right hand between the middle and fourth fingers; the fourth finger of your right hand between the fourth and little fingers; and the middle finger and forefinger of your right hand on the other side of the little finger. Ready to go?

When you are in position push all your fingers as far onto the back of your lover's hand as you can, pushing hard against the back of his hand. Pushing correctly you will have angled the fingers back so that the surface of the palm is stretched taut. Keeping the fingers bent back, stroke the palm with the tips of your thumbs. Press hard. Patiently massage in every tiny crevice. When this stroke is done you will find that all the effort was worth it. It gives credence to the theory that your heart is in your hand.

♡ *Arch Circles*

Oil the sole of the foot. Make a fist with one hand. Steady the foot in your other hand and make slow circles in the arch of the foot. Use firm, deep knuckle pressure. Repeat on the other foot. You can continue this motion to massage all over the bottom of the foot.

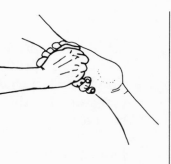

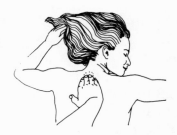

Lovers' Knots

Now place the fingertips of one hand in one of your lover's arches. Place the fingertips of your other hand in one of your lover's palms. Make gentle circles with both your hands on the foot and hand simultaneously. Next move one of your hands to your lover's other hand and make simultaneous circles in both palms. Keep one hand making circles on one of your lover's palms while the other begins circles around one nipple. Continue these light circles all over the body in your own combinations of locations.   Some favorites are: inner thighs and feet; both elbow crooks; backs of knees and elbow crooks; knees and nipples; top of head and navel. For some people, stroking the armpits is erotic. Sensitive and often sensual places to circle and feather include ears, the tip of the nose, the eyelids, the crook of the neck, the wrists, the fingertips and between the toes.

♡ *Full Feathers*

Close the massage with long, light stroking with your fingertips down the full length of the body from head to toe. Trace slightly different paths with each long stoke.

When you've completed a romantic massage, you've exchanged an unforgettable Valentine. An affair full of good massages is a fine romance.

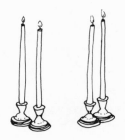

Valentine Celebration

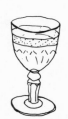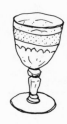

Favorite Wine or Sparkling Grape Juice

Large Prawns and spiced sauce

French Bread and Cambezola Cheese

Salad of sliced melon, rose petals, toasted pine nuts and endive with raspberry vinaigrette

Chocolate-dipped strawberries and orange peel

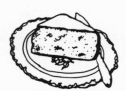

Tantra

During the years that I was teaching Hatha yoga, I also studied a form of Hindu Tantra and a branch of Kundalini yoga which employs fast deep breathing exercises in combination with Hatha postures. Some of these exercises are included in this section because I found they can be helpful for getting in touch with yourself and your partner.

What is unusual to Westerners about Tantric yoga as a spiritual discipline is that it includes sexual energy training. Tantra does not subscribe to a dualistic theory of a split between sensuousness and spirituality, or a theory that views the body as impure.

An informative book of Buddhist Tantra in English is *The Tantric View of Life* by Herbert Guenther (Shambhala, 1970, cloth).

Fulfillment comes through uniting the parts of ourselves and allowing these aspects to fall into their natural balance. All Tantric exercises include a physical and a mental meditation. There is attention to grounding and to the relation of activity and receptivity.

Sexual practices are among the many forms of awareness practices included in Tantra. The sex act (not experienced as relation between subject and object but as a communication between two equal beings) becomes a search for higher integration and the symbol for the uniting of goddess and god.

Non-Looking

Choose a quiet room (or go outdoors) with soft light. Wear nothing or loose fitting clothing. Be sitting opposite but not touching your partner in a comfortable cross-legged position. Let your back be straight but not tense. Relax your hands, palms down, on your knees.

Now look at a spot centered on the bridge of the nose between your partner's eyes. Let your eyes stay with this spot throughout the exercise. If possible do not blink. Allow your breathing to relax, your mind to clear, and your eyes to receive what is in front of them, rather then actively searching out an image. If you feel thoughts beginning to flood your consciousness, allow them to pass right through without focusing on them. Stay receptively focused on that center spot and allow whatever happens visually or emotionally.

Your partner does the same. Do this for about twenty minutes. Now share what the experience was like for both of you.

Palm Circuit

Sit opposite your partner, cross-legged, so that your knees are touching. Relax your breathing. Bend your arms and hold them up in front of you, your palms facing outward about chin high. Place your palms against your partner's palms letting them rest together without straining. Look into each other's eyes and stay with this gaze throughout the exercise.

Do not try to communicate with each other with facial expressions. Allow your eyes to receive without effort. You can do this part of the exercise by itself or add the Breath of Fire.

With short, hard exhalations, pull in your stomach muscles each time you exhale. Now quicken the pace of your breathing, puffing out your abdomen as you inhale and contracting it hard as you exhale, maintaining eye contact. Gradually increase the pace of your breathing until you are breathing as fast as you can through your nose, without sacrificing depth. This is the Breath of Fire.

Stop when the breathing is no longer comfortable. Slow down gradually also. If your arms or back get tired before your breathing, try staying in the position a few moments past the discomfort and the achiness will usually disappear.

Tune in to the feeling of energy inside you, to your partner's energy, and to the current which may be circulating between your bodies through any of your points of contact. Can you relax and allow this energy to flow?

Four Foot Circuit

Straighten out your legs and move apart so that the two of you can sit facing each other with the soles of your feet touching. Let your back be straight but not rigid. Stretch out both arms, shoulder height, in front of you, palms up. Your partner should also stretch his or her arms out toward you, but palms down and slightly above your hands.

Now look into each other's eyes. Maintain this position for about five minutes, tuning in to any energy sensations you might feel moving through your legs, arms and torso.

Now try this with the Breath of Fire.

Back to Back

Sit cross-legged, back to back, with your partner. Try to let as much of your spines touch as possible, especially your lower backs. Find a place to rest together where both of you are comfortable and neither feels too leaned-on or leaning. Extend your arms behind you so that you can comfortably rest your palms on your partner's thighs.

Close your eyes. Tune in to your breathing. Pay attention to any energy sensations moving between your hands and your backs, and especially to the breathing at the base of your spines.

Now try this with the Breath of Fire.

Reichian Massage

Wilhelm Reich used body contact techniques in his work to release deep muscular tension. Described here are two simple exercises for loosening constriction in the thighs, the spine and the pelvis.

Thigh Shake

Be sitting on the floor. Have your partner lie down and rest her left foreleg across your lap so that you can reach her upper thigh muscles without straining. Spread your fingers apart and place one palm on the inside of your partner's thigh, and the other on the outside. Hold her thigh between your hands and shake and vibrate the muscles vigorously. Move and sit beside your partner's right leg and repeat this on the other thigh.

Leg and Hip Release

Your partner lies on the floor on her back. Stand at her feet and grasp her ankles. Slowly raise her two legs lifting from the ankles until both legs are held in the air but the pelvis is still mostly resting on the ground.

Wait in this position a moment until you feel your partner relax and give over the effort of lifting to you. When you have this done to you, try not to tense any of your muscles as your partner lifts. See if you can remain loose while she does the work.

When your partner has released her legs, move your hands palms down onto the soles of her feet. Begin leaning your weight onto your hands and pressing down on the feet. If your partner's legs are relaxed, the knees will bend and be pressed toward her chest. Her pelvis and spine will raise off the floor a bit. If your partner is quite flexible, you will eventually be able to move her knees to the floor over her shoulders. But don't push anyone beyond their flexibility. Move *very* slowly, evenly and gradually. Help her relax and curl up in a ball.

Then, just as slowly and gradually, reverse the movement and lower her legs to the floor again.

You can trade off and have your partner do this to you.

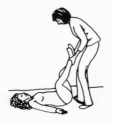 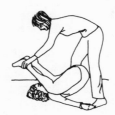

Connecting

Most of us consider only a small portion of our bodies (most likely the pelvic area) erotic. This is a learned adult state different from the natural total responsiveness of a young person's body. "Connecting" is a technique by which you can learn to reopen erotic feelings through your whole body.

While you are touching an area on his body your partner considers highly erotic, with your other hand begin to gently massage an area he considers not particularly sensitive. Massage the two areas simultaneously until your partner reaches a peak of pleasure. Then remove your hand from the first spot while continuing to massage the second. Repeat this sequence several times.

If you do this frequently when you make love or share massage, eventually the newly sensitized areas will become as excitable as the genital or other area.

Talk over with your partner later how he feels about allowing more sensation into this area.

To feel best connecting strokes require covering your partner first with a light film of massage oil. The proportion of how exquisite these strokes feel seems to increase with how light your touch is. The speed will vary some with each individual's taste, but usually should be quite slow.

Your partner lies on his or her back on a bed, massage table, or covered pad on the floor in a warm room.

Sit on your partner's left side facing his or her abdomen. Place both hands, palms down, on the abdomen and begin *very* lightly and *very* slowly making large circles on this area with your whole hand. Continue these circles for a while.

Now slowly separate your hands, moving one palm down the inside of your partner's leg and the other up the chest. Your right hand moving across the chest traces a line from the abdomen, across the ribs, over the left nipple, over the left pectoral muscle arc, and into the armpit. *At the same time* your left hand moves from the abdomen, over the hip, down the inside of the thigh, inside the calf, across the ankle, ending up in the arch of your partner's left foot.

Much of the success of this stroke depends on timing: your hands should be crossing the thigh and ribs at the same time and should also reach the armpit and foot arch simultaneously. Now, make slow *light* circles in each arch with your two hands in time; stay with this light motion a while.

Now begin the return trip. Retrace your paths toward the abdomen, moving still slowly and feather lightly. (Cross the thigh and side simultaneously.) End with a few more circles on the abdomen.

Repeat this stroke on your partner's right side.

Two V's

Your partner is lying on his or her back. You will need to be sitting, facing toward your partner's head, about parallel to his or her left knee. Place both hands on the left foot. Position your hands so that your thumbs and fingers form a V cupping the top of the foot. Move slowly and lightly. At first move both hands together side by side over the ankle and onto the calf.

Now pace your outer (right) hand faster than your inside hand (because you want your right hand to reach the armpit when the inside hand reaches your partner's crotch). The path of your right hand is up the outside of your partner's left leg, over the hip, over the abdomen and ribs and left nipple, until your fingers are on the left pectoral muscles.

All the while your left hand has been moving even more slowly up the inside of your partner's left leg so that your fingers touch the crease between the thigh and the pelvis *just as* your upper hand touches the crease of the armpit. Now

137

your two hands are going to simultaneously do the same light squeezing stroke. Do this by moving both sets of fingertips simultaneously down the crease of the armpit and the crease of the pelvis. As your thumbs slide toward your fingers in this motion, "pinch" thumbs and forefingers together lightly as they move down the two creases. Particularly pleasing about this stroke is the "rolling" sensation created by the repetition of stroking the two areas, once with your fingers and again with your thumbs—and the internal sensation that the two areas being massaged are somehow the same.

Now quite slowly retrace the path of both hands down your partner's left side, ending as you began with both palms resting on the foot. Repeat the stroke on your partner's right side.

Other Connections

You can also try inventing your own strokes for connecting: the mouth and the nipples, the perineum and the back of the neck, the mouth and the genitals, the palms of the hands and the bottom centers of the feet, the anus and the bottom centers of your feet, the tip of the nose and the nipples.

Sensate Focus

In their studies of human sexual behavior, Drs. Johnson and Masters found that the inhibitions of rigid role behavior are a major block to sexual pleasure. An exercise they offer for opening up some of these behaviors is called Sensate Focus.

The aims of Sensate Focus are to give each partner a chance to experience being totally aggressive sexually, and then also totally receptive; and to free your sexual activity from time clocks and goals.

Choose a time when you both feel relaxed and unhurried and will not be interrupted. The basic activity of Sensate Focus is massage so the room you use should be comfortably warm for both of you to be nude.

If you are usually the more receptive and responsive of the two of you in lovemaking, it is your turn to take the aggressive role. After a hot bath or shower, have your partner lie face down on a massage table, the bed, or a pad on the floor covered with a sheet. Spread warm oil all over your partner's body and then begin to massage the feet. Work extremely slowly and intricately. *Don't worry about technical strokes.* You are touching your partner to communicate your feelings, not your expertise. Do what your hands want to. You can include lots of feather light stroking along with firm smooth strokes with your palms and fingers. Work your way slowly up the legs and back.

Now have your partner turn over. Massage from the feet up the legs slowly to the hips. Bypass the genitals and massage the stomach, chest and face.

It is important as you do this that both of you have a desire to forget about time and the "goal" of orgasm. If you are receiving, let yourself be massaged without directing it and get into the current feelings you are having in whatever part of your body is being touched. If you can do this you will discover new areas and dimensions of pleasure. Paradoxically also, if you do have an orgasm, it will be fuller and more powerful for your having allowed relaxation and more feeling to flow into every part of your body.

Finally as the giver of the massage you do massage the pelvic areas and the genitals. By now your partner is probably feeling extremely relaxed and sensitized so that your lightest touch on the genital area will be felt. Massage all the intricate contours of your partner's genitals very slowly and carefully and gently. Now and then use one of your hands to massage another area of your partner's body simultaneously. If you had agreed at the beginning of the massage to continue until orgasm, keep massaging the particularly erotic areas until your partner is satisfied. Try to be open and responsive to your partner's individual rhythm. If you are receiving the massage try to see what happens if you let yourself relax and go completely *at your own pace* without any thought of hurrying for someone else or pleasing them.

Afterward share your feelings about how the massage was to give and receive. On another day, trade places and be the receiver while your partner is the giver. In which role are you more comfortable?

Genital Push-ups

Drs. Johnson and Masters give women vaginal exercises to do daily to increase genital strength and feeling. The exercises are extremely simple and can be done often and anywhere. No one will know!

The muscles women are interested in contracting for this exercise are called the pubococcygeal muscles, or pelvic floor. (Feel them working by trying to stop your urine in mid-flow the next time you urinate.) Do this several times and you will get a sense of how to contract these muscles. Contract and release the muscles alternately, slowly at about the speed and rhythm of the *Blue Danube Waltz*. Try to really contract the muscles and pull up so that you begin to get some sense of the connected muscles inside the pelvis.

This is an important set of muscles because it forms the "pelvic floor" which supports your organs when you stand. Flexibility in this area is very important during sex, pregnancy and childbirth. The more these muscles are exercised, the more feeling and awareness develops in them, the more pleasure you will be able to feel.

140

The variation for men simply involves contracting and releasing the muscles of the groin in the same pattern.

Push Outs

Use these same muscles at the same slow pace as in the exercise above. Alternate contracting and pushing out in the area, but this time emphasize the pushing out part of the cycle. Experiment with this during sex and in other situations too.

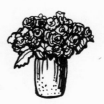

Body Techniques for Increasing Orgasm in Women

> Masters and Johnson position: the woman sits in front of partner between his or her legs, leaning back and resting on their chest. Her partner uses a warm oil or cream to massage her torso, and then genitals.

Hatha yoga

Breathing relaxation techniques

Massage

Connecting

Knowledge of own and partner's anatomy

Vaginal push-ups

Masturbation

Clearly communicating what you want and like

Body Techniques To Help Men Prolong Erection

Rhythmical contraction and release of the muscles of the genital area, about 50 times, once a day

Any kind of exercise, or more especially yoga, which improves general body condition *without* creating a muscle-bound condition

Knowledge of male and female anatomy

Masturbation (once or twice a week) to the point of—*but without*—ejaculation

Massage

Masters and Johnson Sensate Focus

The Oriental technique of squeezing each testicle once for every year of your life, once a day

Clearly communicating what you want and like

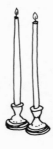

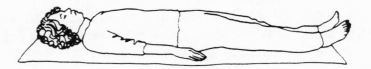

The Basic Breath

The Basic Breath can be used for healing, to increase circulation in an area, to speed up tissue regeneration after injury, to relieve pain. It can also be used to heighten sensitivity in an area. But its main purpose is to be a means of bringing you to the state of your own natural breathing rhythm. The Basic Breath exercise was developed by Magdalene Proskauer, a San Francisco therapist who specialized in analyzing the psychological aspects of breathing.

There are different exercises for each part of the body, but the same three-part breath is used in all of them. This breathing cycle is designed to trigger your natural rhythm gradually. By using this cycle you can let go of imposed rhythms and allow your own to surface. When in a couple relationship, most of us have to struggle to maintain a clear identity without getting it mixed up with that of our partner. The Basic Breath exercise offers you a means of finding your center, your deepest sense of yourself no matter what is going on around you.

Lie on your back on the bed or floor. Relax your arms at your sides and let your feet fall out to the sides. Close your eyes and feel the way you are lying on the floor. Notice whether any part of your body feels a bit tense or doesn't seem to be resting comfortably on the surface beneath you. Now move your focus inside your body and notice where you feel movement as you breathe.

If you feel tense anywhere, try imagining that you can breathe into the tension, as though you could actually exhale through that body part. Imagine the breath relaxing your sore muscle as it moves through it. Breathing into a body part is something you can do anywhere, any time you feel tense or nervous. Locate the tight place and "breathe into it." Breathe in sync with the tensing (inhale) and relaxing (exhale) of your movement.

As you are doing this exercise, loosen your clothing if it is tight at the waist. Let the muscles of your stomach and abdomen relax and let your breath sink lower in your body. Place one hand palm down at the lowest place on your torso where you can feel the motion of your breathing. Now let your hand and arm relax at your side again. If you see any pictures of yourself or other images during this breathing exercise, remember them and draw or write them down later.

Relax your jaw and open your mouth a little so that you can exhale through your mouth. You don't need to breathe heavily. Relax and breathe naturally. Inhale through your nose; exhale through your mouth; and pause at the end of the exhalation before you breathe again. This pause is the key to the effectiveness of the breathing. Crucial things are happening to your body during the pause; you are actually still exhaling, though you may feel as though nothing is going on. Deepening your exhalation gets all the stale air out of your lungs, and makes more room for fresh air when you inhale. Most of us don't exhale deeply enough. Often, when you feel that you can't take in enough air, and that you'd like to inhale more deeply, it's because you haven't exhaled fully enough to make room in your lungs for new air. This is usually the breathing difficulty in asthma. Lengthening your exhalation can help release asthmatic symptoms.

You have paused at the end of the exhalation for a long time now. Let yourself really explore the pause. How does it feel to you? Does it feel too long? Not long enough? Are you a little worried that your body won't breathe in again unless you make it? Think of your breathing when you are asleep. You don't have to tell yourself to breathe then. Think of animals breathing when they are resting. Their breath is long and rolling. They don't tell themselves to breathe. You can learn to trust that your breath will always come in again.

Allow the pause to be as long as it wants. It may feel very long. See whether you can wait and stay with the pause until your body wants to breathe in again by itself. Inhale through your nose; exhale through your mouth; then pause and wait. It's a little like standing on the beach and waiting for another wave to come in. Try to find a pace at which you are neither holding your breath to prolong the pause nor making yourself breathe in again. Let yourself breathe in this pattern as long as you want.

This exercise in itself is deeply relaxing. If you have difficulty going to sleep, you can use this breath at night. Or any time you feel tense you can take a few minutes off for yourself, relax, and find your rhythm again.

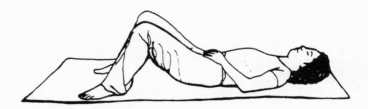

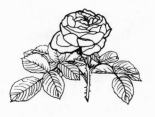

Diary

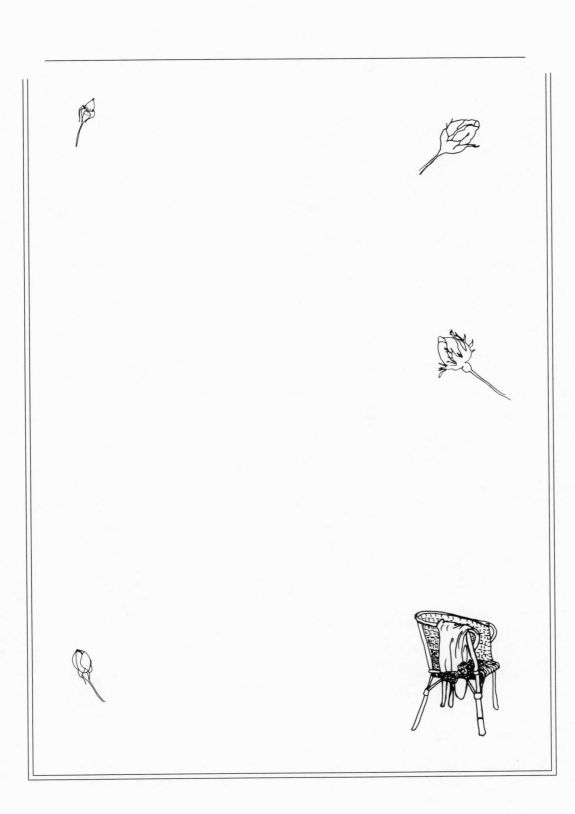

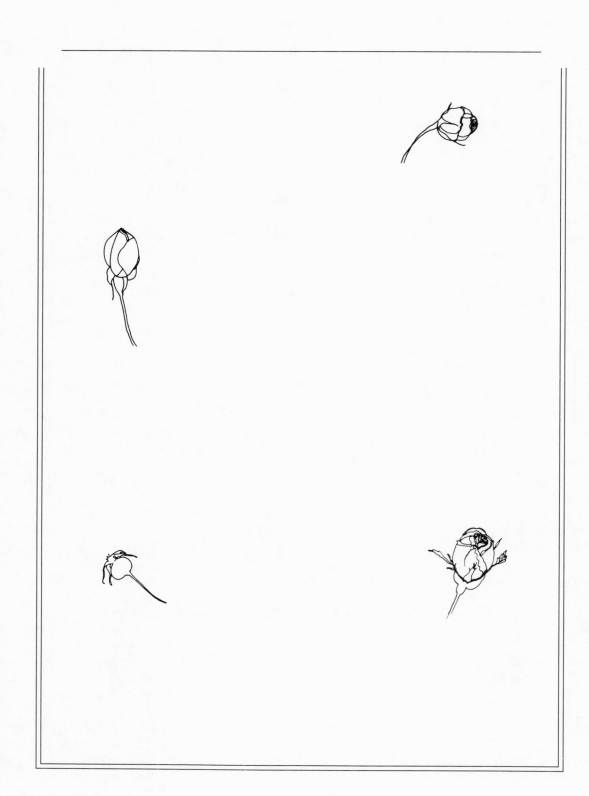

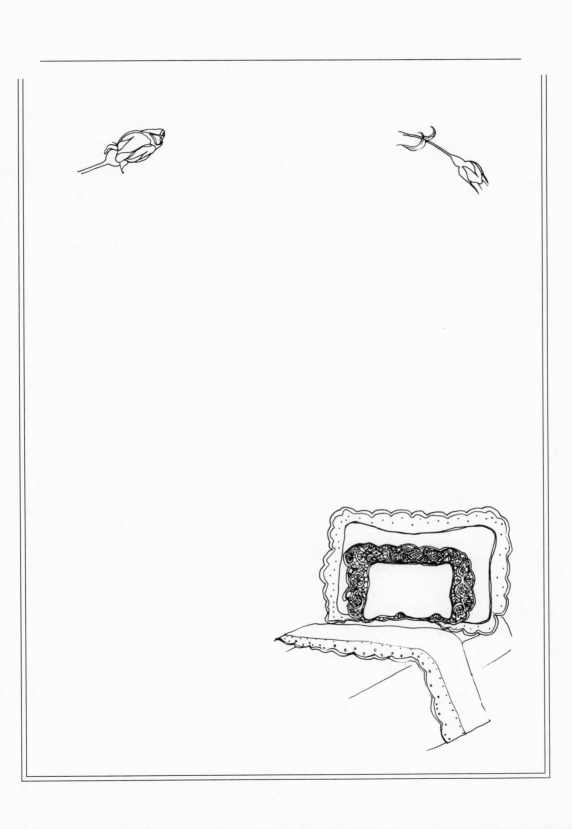

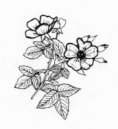

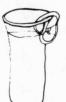

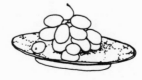

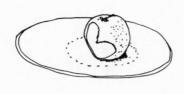

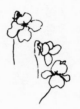

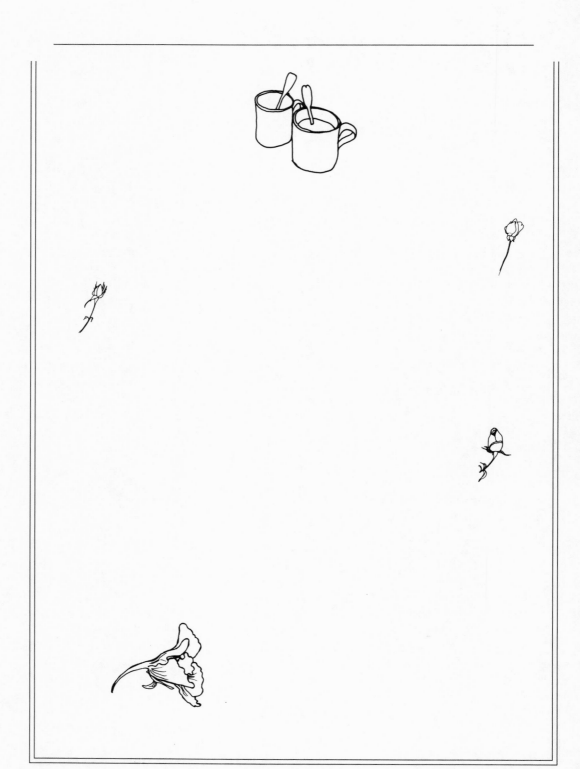

Roses in Order of Appearance

Rosa alba Regalis

Rosa Canina Burboniana

Rosa Rubifolia

Rosa alba Regalis

Rosa Damascena aurora

Rosa Gallica Versicolor

Rosa Indica Vulgaris

Rosa Berberifolia

Rosa flore submultiplici

Rosa Pumila

Rosa Indica fragrans

Rosa Camanulata alba

Rosa Noisettiana

Rosa bifera officinalis

Rosa Indica Pumila

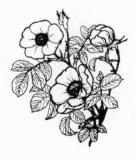

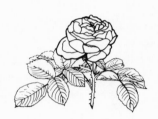

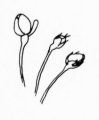

The Author

Anne Kent Rush, a descendant of Dr. Benjamin Rush, an American health revolutionary who signed the Declaration of Independence, was born in Mobile, Alabama. She is the author of *The Back Rub Book; Getting Clear: Body Work for Women; Moon, Moon; The Basic Back Book;* co-author of *Feminism as Therapy;* and illustrator of *The Massage Book.* Rush was on the training staffs of Alyssum Center and of Esalen Institute in California, was a partner in Moon Books, and has taught in the U. S. and Europe. She wrote and illustrated *Greta Bear Goes to Yellowstone National Park,* the first in a series of children's travel books on wildlife conservation.

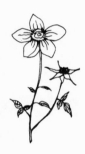

Avon Books are available at special quantity discounts for bulk purchases for sales promotions, premiums, fund raising or educational use. Special books, or book excerpts, can also be created to fit specific needs.

For details write or telephone the office of the Director of Special Markets, Avon Books, Dept. FP, 105 Madison Avenue, New York, New York 10016; 212-481-5653.

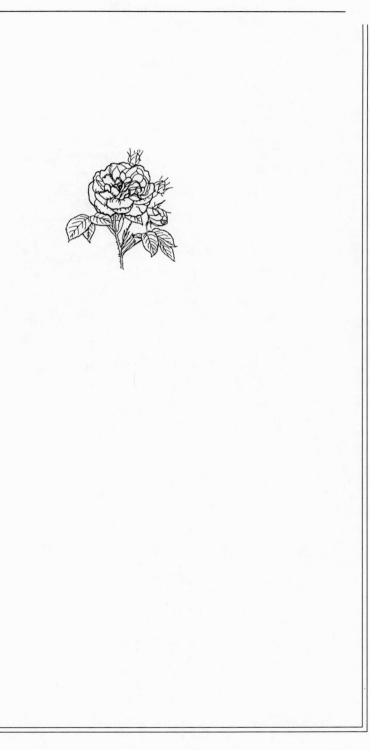

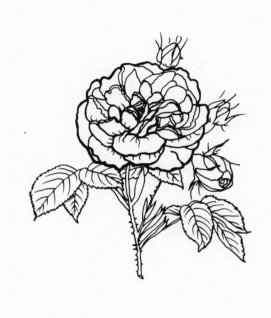